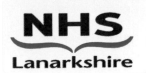

THE FUTURE HEALTH WORKER

by Liz Kendall and
Rachel Lissauer

30-32 Southampton Street, London WC2E 7RA
Tel: 020 7470 6100 Fax: 020 7470 6111
info@ippr.org
www.ippr.org
Registered charity 800065

The Institute for Public Policy Research (ippr), established in 1988, is Britain's leading independent think tank on the centre left. The values that drive our work include delivering social justice, deepening democracy, increasing environmental sustainability and enhancing human rights. Through our well-researched and clearly argued policy analysis, our publications, our media events, our strong networks in government, academia and the corporate and voluntary sector, we play a vital role in maintaining the momentum of progressive thought.

ippr's aim is to bridge the political divide between the social democratic and liberal traditions, the intellectual divide between the academics and the policy makers and the cultural divide between the policy-making establishment and the citizen. As an independent institute, we have the freedom to determine our research agenda. ippr has charitable status and is funded by a mixture of corporate, charitable, trade union and individual donations.

Research is ongoing, and new projects being developed, in a wide range of policy areas including sustainability, health and social care, social policy, citizenship and governance, education, economics, democracy and community, media and digital society and public private partnerships. In future we aim to grow into a permanent centre for contemporary progressive thought, recognised both at home and globally.

For further information you can contact ippr's external affairs department on info@ippr.org, you can view our website at www.ippr.org and you can buy our books from Central Books on 0845 458 9910 or email ippr@centralbooks.com.

Production & design by **EMPHASIS**
ISBN 1 86030 214 9
© IPPR 2003

Contents

Acknowledgements

We would like to thank the sponsors of the Future Health Worker project – Boots the Chemists, Pfizer, PRIME and Lloydspharmacy – without whose generous support this book would not have been possible.

We are grateful to the members of the Future Health Worker Advisory Group for all their help and advice throughout the course of the project. They include: Howard Catton, Royal College of Nursing; Sir Cyril Chantler, Great Ormond Street Hospital; Paul Chapman, UNISON; Nigel Edwards, NHS Confederation; Pippa Gough, King's Fund; Judy Hargadon, Department of Health Changing Workforce Programme; Mike Pringle, University of Nottingham; Jane Salvage, Author and Health Consultant and Sian Williams, Independent Management Consultant. However, the views expressed in this report remain the responsibility of the authors alone.

We are also grateful to the authors of the papers which formed the basis of the project's seminar series, and to the contributors to the interim publication of the Future Health Worker project: *New practitioners in the future health service: exploring roles for practitioners in primary and intermediate care.*

Finally, we would like to thank all those who gave their time to comment on earlier drafts of this report, particularly Jane Naish, Peter Robinson, Matthew Taylor and Lisa Harker, and Helena Scott for all her valuable help in producing this report.

About the authors

Liz Kendall is an Associate Director at IPPR and responsible for running the Institute's programme of research on health and social care. She was previously the Fellow of the Public Health Programme at the King's Fund. From 1996 to 1998, Liz was a Special Adviser to the Rt Hon Harriet Harman MP, Secretary of State for Social Security and Minister for Women. Her most recent publications include *An Equal Start? Improving support during pregnancy and the first twelve months* (2003), *From Welfare to Wellbeing: the future of social care* (2002) and *The Future Patient* (2001).

Rachel Lissauer is the Surgery Improvement Manager at the Mayday Healthcare NHS Trust. She was previously a Research Fellow in Health Policy at the IPPR and led the work of the Future Health Worker project. Prior to this, Rachel was a member of the secretariat for IPPR's Commission on Public Private Partnerships where she carried out the Commission's work on PPPs in health and education. Her previous publications include: *New practitioners in the future health service: exploring roles for practitioners in primary and intermediate care* (2002); *Building Better Partnerships* (2001); *PPPs in Primary Care* (2000) and *A Learning Process: PPPs in education* (2000).

Executive summary

Introduction

NHS staff play a critical role in delivering a more socially just society. However, the historically lower levels of spending on, and lower proportion of staff employed by, the NHS compared to healthcare systems in other European countries mean too many health workers have to struggle to provide care in difficult and challenging circumstances.

The pressures facing the health workforce are set to increase in future. A more informed and educated population and the decline in deference means clinicians are questioned in ways unimaginable twenty years ago. New information technologies are transforming the way health services are delivered and scientific advances are expanding our knowledge about the causes and pathways of disease.

NHS staff have not been immune to these developments. Their working practices, attitudes and cultures have undergone substantial changes in recent years. However, there is much further to travel before the health workforce is ready to meet the demands of a 21st century healthcare system. Too many clinicians fail to share information and control with patients, treating them as passive recipients rather than equal partners in their own treatment and care. Professional organisations and trades unions often remain pre-occupied with protecting their members' interests and identities, instead of promoting the patient's interest or improving working relations with other members of the healthcare team. Restrictive practices and entrenched professional hierarchies can still work against the development of sufficiently flexible and responsive services.

Reforming the health workforce presents major challenges for progressive politics. The invaluable contribution health professionals make must be better recognised whilst simultaneously questioning whether these professions require fundamental reform. Professional hierarchies and working practices which prevent the delivery of patient-centred care must be tackled, without belittling the commitment and sacrifices made by those same professions every day of their working lives.

Pre-occupation with structural reform

The NHS employs 1.25 million people; the social care sector a similar number. Between them, health and social care services employ one in ten of the UK working population. Staff costs account for around two thirds of all NHS expenditure. Without the right number of people, with the right skills, in the right locations, the NHS will fail to deliver high quality, comprehensive care over the coming years.

Whilst successive governments have talked about the need to give priority to reforming working practices, their overwhelming focus has been on structural change. Yet the evidence that reforming NHS structures has led to improved outcomes for patients is hard to come by. In addition, most practitioners regard structural change as irrelevant to their daily work. Research suggests only one in five clinicians are aware of any major structural changes since 1997. Those that are regard these changes as having little if any relevance for the way in which they provide care.

One reason for the preoccupation with structural reform is that past attempts to change working practices have proved difficult and controversial. In particular, doctors have opposed the perceived encroachment on their professional autonomy by politicians, through their proxy at the local level - the health service manager. This was one of the main factors behind the rejection of the consultant contract in England and Wales.

A sense of disengagement with the process of reform now exists amongst many clinicians. There is a profound contrast between the responsibility staff feel for providing patient care and the degree of power and influence they believe they can exert over 'the system'. Addressing this problem is one of the most important issues facing the NHS and will be critical to the success of future workforce reforms.

The need for a coherent vision

Professional organisations, trades unions and government all agree that further changes to working practices will be required in the years ahead. Yet there is little agreement about what the overall shape of the future health workforce should look like.

The objective of any workforce reform must be to improve the quality of care being provided so that it better meets the needs of patients and improves patient outcomes. This goal is one that politicians, practitioners and patients alike can support and around which consensus for change can be built.

However in order to make this goal more than a superficial aspiration, a much clearer and more precise definition of what high quality, patient-centred care is must be developed. Whilst the term 'patient-centred care' is frequently used, its precise meaning can differ according to who uses it. Professional bodies often automatically conflate their members' interests with those of patients, when this may not necessarily be the case. The Government's definition of patient-centred care is primarily about making access to services more timely and convenient and improving patients' choices about where and when their operations take place. Whilst these are certainly important features of a patient-centred system, they do not amount to a sufficiently broad or far sighted definition of the term.

Defining 'patient-centred' care

Patient-centred care must be based on an understanding of what patients want from their health services, but also on the evidence of what is necessary to deliver better patient outcomes. It should provide a framework for improving current services but also seek to anticipate relevant future trends.

High quality, patient-centred care can be summarised by five broad characteristics:

- Safe and effective

- Promoting health and wellbeing

- Integrated and seamless

- Informing and empowering

- Timely and convenient.

Where workforce reforms have taken place, they have tended to focus on short term goals such as improving patient safety and making access to services more timely and convenient. Far less attention has been paid to how workforce reforms might contribute to equally important characteristics of patient-centred care such as promoting and restoring health and informing and empowering patients. More fundamental changes to the workforce will therefore be necessary in order to deliver genuinely patient-centred care in future.

Safe and effective

Patients should not be harmed by the care that is intended to help them. Care that is unsafe can not only harm individual patients but also make the overall health system less cost-effective. Serious failures in practice are uncommon relative to the high volume of care that is provided. There is nevertheless worrying evidence about the rates of serious medical failures in the NHS. Estimates suggest that adverse events in which harm is caused to patients occur in around ten per cent of admissions.

Patients should also receive care which is based on the best available evidence. Evidence-based practice requires those who give care to consistently avoid both under-use of effective care and over-use of ineffective care. Research suggests that around a fifth of interventions in areas like general medicine and general practice are not evidence-based.

Barriers to change

Professional values, cultures and working practices have had an important impact on the safety and effectiveness of healthcare being provided. There are also system-wide barriers to delivering safe health care (as highlighted by the Bristol Royal Infirmary Inquiry) and effective health care (it has been estimated that doctors would need to read 19 articles a day, 365 days a year to keep up to speed with 'evidence-based' practice).

Recent changes

A wide range of initiatives are being implemented to ensure individual practitioners and the NHS as a whole deliver safer, more effective patient care. A mandatory, national reporting scheme for adverse healthcare events and near misses in the NHS is being established alongside a new independent National Patient Safety Agency. A range of mechanisms are being used to set and monitor standards across the NHS including National Service Frameworks, the National Institute for Clinical Excellence and the Commission for Healthcare Audit and Inspection. Inter-professional training is being introduced to ensure more open and effective team working. The new Council for the Regulation of Healthcare Professionals is intended to strengthen and co-ordinate the system of professional self-regulation, and revalidation and appraisal for doctors is being introduced to help improve standards. An Electronic Library for Health is also being established to support clinicians in adopting evidence based practice.

Future challenges

Many of these developments are still at an early stage and their impact will be hard to determine for some while. However, several challenges for the future are already apparent. These include transforming pre- and post- qualification education to ensure clinicians have the necessary skills to deliver safe and effective care; addressing the practical and cultural barriers to implementing inter-professional training; ensuring non-professionally qualified staff do not remain entirely un-regulated in future; and assessing the impact on safety and effectiveness of the likely shift towards more care being delivered in primary care and in patients' homes.

Promoting health and wellbeing

Genuinely patient-centred care not only effectively treats illness but also seeks to prevent ill health and promote good health. Preventing people from becoming ill so they do not have to go to hospital for more invasive and potentially dangerous procedures, and rehabilitating older people so they can live independently rather than remaining in hospital or in a care home, are important goals not only because they are likely to improve patient satisfaction but because they will lead to better health outcomes and improved cost-effectiveness across the system as a whole.

Lack of priority for public health

The current Government, in stark contrast to the previous one, has acknowledged the existence of health inequalities and their close relationship with social and economic factors. However, the overwhelming focus of policy is still on improving health care rather than improving health. Whilst national health inequality targets have been set, they do not have real 'bite' compared to key performance indicators such as targets to improve waiting times; and whilst Primary Care Trusts have been given a mandate to improve the health of their local population, the enormity of the task they face in both commissioning and providing health services means public health is inevitably a secondary concern.

Medical model of health

The reasons for the focus on treating ill health, rather than promoting or restoring good health, are complex. The power and control traditionally afforded to doctors within the health system and the dominance of a medical model of health has been a major factor, exerting a powerful influence on the way health practitioners work, how they relate to one another, and their relationships with patients and local communities.

The short-termism of the political system has also played an important role: politicians need to show results within the course of an electoral cycle whilst the benefits of upstream interventions to prevent ill health may not be seen for many years. In addition, the media tends to give greater prominence to stories of 'miracle' cures or patients left waiting on trolleys in Accident and Emergency departments, than to research or initiatives which demonstrate prevention is better than cure.

Impact on practitioners and patients

Medicine has had a hugely beneficial impact on the lives of millions of patients. Every year new advances bring the ability to cure previously untreatable diseases.

However, the dominance of the medical model of health has sometimes had less positive consequences for patient care. It has been an important factor behind the greater status (and resources) attached to specialist services provided in hospitals than to other forms of care. It has also resulted in a lack of resources and priority being given to public health skills. The so-called 'Cinderella' services that use teams of practitioners to deliver care within communities, like mental health and social care, are seen as less prestigious or interesting and offer few merit awards and little private practice. The tendency to 'medicalise' health problems could accelerate in future: drugs which seek to treat problems which have previously been regarded as non-medical are already on the market and more are set to emerge in the years ahead. Addressing the dominance of the medical model of health and giving greater prominence to public health priorities and skills is a major challenge for the NHS and its workforce.

Integrated and seamless

Patient-centred care effectively co-ordinates services within the NHS and between the NHS and other sectors like social care. However, quantitative and qualitative research of patients' experiences suggests there are major difficulties in delivering fully integrated services across all parts of the system. UK patients appear more likely to experience difficulties in the co-ordination of services than those in other countries.

Increasing specialisation

The sheer number of different staff involved in the process of care presents major challenges to effective co-ordination. This problem is exacerbated by the increasing specialisation of the health workforce. Whilst the value of specialist care must not be underestimated, it may also come at a price: a lack of investment in generalist skills and the poor co-ordination of services. Finding an appropriate balance between specialist and generalist skills is a key issue facing all health care systems in future.

Clarifying roles, developing new practitioners

Another factor which can inhibit the delivery of seamless services is the lack of clarity about who does what in the process of care. Evaluations of local collaborative programmes, which seek to clarify the patients' pathway through the system, indicate significant improvements in the quality of patient care. Ensuring clinicians feel ownership over the process of change is critical to the success of these initiatives.

The need to improve co-ordination between different members of the health workforce and to clarify roles is an important factor behind the drive towards inter-professional training. It has also led to new types of workers whose skills cut across traditional professional divides being developed in the non-professionally qualified workforce. It has been argued that a radical simplification and streamlining of the professional as well as support workforce will be critical in delivering more patient centred care in future.

Changing working practices

The difficulties of integrating health and social care services are well known. Poor co-ordination has been repeatedly identified as a major failing in the system, particularly in relation to older people's services. The Government's main response to this problem is to propose further structural change, for example through the development of Care Trusts. Yet the evidence that structural change improves the integration of health and social care services at the front line is far from persuasive.

Better outcomes for those with health and social care needs may well be achieved by changing working practices, rather than by further structural reform. Greater use of integrated care pathways, based on evidence-based protocols which specify the roles, responsibilities and sequence of interventions by the different professionals involved will be crucial. New types of practitioners who combine health and social care roles that are currently separate may also need to emerge, such as new intermediate care practitioners who provide rehabilitation services for older people.

Informing and empowering

One of the most important challenges facing the NHS is the need to provide for patients more and better quality information. Patients suffer from poor communication and a lack of information in all health care systems, but this may be a particular problem in the UK. Whilst today's patients don't get enough information, tomorrow's may suffer the opposite problem because of the explosion of information available over the internet.

Empowering patients is not simply about providing patients with more and better quality information: it is also about ensuring that those patients who want to can use information to participate in decisions about their own treatment and care. Sharing decisions with patients can lead to better outcomes, reduced anxiety and depression, and improved satisfaction rates. The Government has recognised the need to encourage patients to take on greater roles, for example through the Expert Patient programme. However, only £3 million has been invested in the initiative so far – a drop in the ocean compared to the scale of the task at hand.

Changing attitudes

Professional attitudes, particularly those of doctors, have been an important barrier to informing and empowering patients in the past. Being the sole possessor of a unique body of knowledge and expertise has been at the heart of doctors' sense of professionalism. This belief is being increasingly challenged as patients become more educated and informed. Many – although not all – doctors now recognise they are no longer the only creators or custodians of health information.

Doctors' failure to communicate effectively with patients is also related to patients' reluctance to share the risks and problems associated with medicine and healthcare, as well as its potential benefits. In future, patients' roles will need to evolve as much as doctors'. Patients need to understand the limits to modern medicine, as well as its capacity to bring about change.

It is important to recognise the system-wide barriers to informing and empowering patients. Research suggests that 20 minute consultations are needed to effectively involve patients in decisions about treatment, give them a sense of control and enable them to take on responsibility for some aspects of their care. Yet time is a rare commodity in the NHS – something which is keenly felt by patients and professionals alike.

New skills for practitioners

The process of informing patients, involving them in decisions and sharing risks is highly complex. Some patients will want more involvement and information than others. Patients' preferences are likely to change over time, and depend on a range of factors such as their age and clinical condition.

Practitioners will need a range of skills to work effectively with patients in future. Communication skills are becoming a core part of undergraduate training for every new health professional. However, concerns about the effectiveness of this training have already been raised. Research suggests that educators tend to focus on training doctors to 'tell' patients facts, rather than on enabling patients to act as partners in the process of care. Improving the communication skills of existing professionals remains a considerable challenge.

Patient-professional contracts

New ways of shaping patient-professional relationships may be required in addition to changes in professional training. 'Contracts' between patients and doctors could be developed in future. These might take the shape of a general understanding, but could also follow a more concrete form, involving a specific set of rights and responsibilities negotiated between patients, their doctors and other members of the health team. Such a contract might be particularly appropriate for patients with long-term conditions, since their role in the process of care is integral to improving health outcomes.

Timely and convenient

The speed with which health services can be accessed is a key priority for patients and one of the main sources of dissatisfaction with the NHS. Patients also want more flexible services to fit in with work and family responsibilities.

Providing quicker, more convenient services is therefore vital to improving patient satisfaction. Timely services also play an important role in improving health outcomes and ensuring the overall cost-effectiveness of system: if access to healthcare is inappropriately delayed and a patient's condition worsens, or if patients end up in Accident and Emergency departments because they cannot access timely services in primary care, then health services may be both less clinically and cost-effective.

A publicly funded service must seek to respond to the changing aspirations of the society it seeks to serve if it is to retain sufficient support over the long term. However, the NHS is not just another consumer organisation: it is a public service with a different purpose and set of objectives. Encouraging patients to view the NHS from a purely consumerist perspective will lead to inevitable dissatisfaction since there will always be difficult trade-offs between the needs of individual patients and those of the wider community.

Increasing capacity

Reducing waiting times means increasing capacity in the NHS, and getting more staff into the system is crucial to achieving this goal. The Government has made considerable progress in this area, particularly on its targets to increase the number of nurses. However several trends, such as the ageing workforce and the falling number of applicants to medical school, suggest that increasing the capacity of the NHS workforce in future will depend as much on changing the roles and responsibilities of health workers as on increasing their overall number.

Changing roles

Staff shortages, combined with changing staff aspirations, have led to many practitioners extending their scope of practice over recent years.

Nurses have taken on a range of extra roles and responsibilities. They are increasingly acting as the 'first port of call' in the NHS, for example assessing and giving advice to patients with minor conditions through NHS Direct and Walk in Centres. Many nurse prescribers and nurse practitioners are based in primary care and nurses are also leading a number of Primary Medical Service (PMS) pilot schemes. Research demonstrates that the expansion of nurses' roles has helped deliver higher levels of patient satisfaction and a quality of care that is at least as good as, if not better than, that provided by doctors.

Other practitioners are also taking on new roles. 'Specialist interest' GPs are providing access to services previously only available in secondary care. An extension of prescribing rights means that pharmacists will be able to prescribe a wider range of medicines on the basis of guidelines developed in conjunction with doctors. The roles of physiotherapists and occupational therapists, paramedics and surgical assistants are also evolving.

Insufficient focus on primary care

Whilst there have been changes in the working practices of staff across the health sector, there has tended to be a greater focus on developing roles in secondary care, rather than in primary care or across health and social care. This is for a number of reasons, including the generally higher priority given to healthcare policy in the acute sector, the higher costs associated with staff in secondary care, and the fact that GPs have traditionally exerted considerable influence over developments in staff roles in primary care. There has also been a greater focus on expanding the roles of nurses than other members of the healthcare team. However, if nurses themselves become 'overburdened', the benefits to patients may become less clear. The relationship between nurses and the non-professionally qualified workforce will be brought to the fore in future.

Barriers to change

Professional attitudes have proved an important barrier to changing staff roles to date. For example, evaluations of nurse-led PMS schemes found that whilst some medics 'championed' nurses taking on bigger roles, others were less supportive. Nurse practitioners reported that consultants were sceptical about their referrals, sometimes refusing to accept them. Consultants' attitudes have also been an important barrier to changing GPs' roles: for example, whilst some consultants have welcomed the development of Specialist GPs, others say they feel strongly that GPSIs promote 'second class' care.

A lack of support from professional organisations has been another barrier to change. Nurse practitioners have reported a lack of training and support for their new roles from relevant professional bodies in the past. Legal and practical barriers, such as restricted powers of prescription or certification have also proved problematic. Restrictions on nurses' roles in the UK contrast with the USA, where nurse practitioners practise without any requirement for physician supervision or collaboration in 50 per cent of States.

Future challenges

Future developments (like new diagnostic and monitoring equipment and telemedicine) herald the possibility of more health care being delivered in patients' homes. The expectations of professionals and patients could move from a presumption that inpatient treatment is the norm to the view that patients should be treated in their own home wherever possible. At its boldest, this may result in a 'home first' standard where all health services are delivered in the patient's normal place of residence unless certain factors apply.

A new 'rule' of continuous access to information, care and support, 24 hours a day, 365 days a year could also be developed in future. This would not necessarily imply more visits to see health practitioners, but better use of different means of communicating with patients for example by e-mail and telephone, and better provision of health information ranging from patients' medical records to information about conditions and treatments.

This new vision for accessing health care will require major changes to pre-registration and continuing education for practitioners, greater investment in and support for Information Technology in the NHS, and much closer integration of the health and social care workforce.

The way forward

The working practices, cultures and attitudes of health practitioners are critical in determining the quality of care that is provided. Any government which seeks to improve the quality of health services must make reforming the health workforce a priority in future. Four key challenges are now clear.

- *Improving relations between clinicians and managers.* The evidence shows that the key to successfully reforming working practices is engaging clinicians, particularly doctors, and demonstrating direct improvements to patient care. Measures must be taken to more effectively involve clinicians in managing the process of reform at all levels of the NHS.

- *Ensuring closer working between practitioners and sectors.* Many of the key features of patient-centred care rely on closer working between different members of the health team. This suggests that a shift in culture towards a new professionalism, based on shared practice, knowledge and values is required, in contrast to the traditional model of professionalism which emphasises the differences between professions through seperate systems of regulation, pay and education.

- *Transforming practitioner-patient relations.* Practitioners must not only effectively inform and involve patients in treatment decisions, but also enable them to take on appropriate responsibilities for their own wellbeing and care. This will require major changes in the roles of practitioners and patients alike.

- *Addressing the dominance of the medical model of health.* Patient centred-care must seek to prevent ill health, and promote and restore good health as well as treat illness and disease. It must take a whole person perspective, addressing people's social and emotional needs as well as their physical and medical ones.

Transforming training

Future health workers will need a range of new skills in order to deliver genuinely patient centred care. These include the ability to find new knowledge as it continually expands and to incorporate it into practice; to understand the root causes of ill health and disease, and the relationship between an individual patient's needs and those of the wider community; to work collaboratively in teams, with shared responsibilities for patient care; to adopt a shared decision making approach to patient professional interactions, for those patients who want it; to support patients to take on appropriate responsibilities for their health and care, including how to self-care for minor conditions and self-manage long term illnesses; and to understand managers' roles and the contribution they make to patient care, rather than solely focusing on the individual clinical intervention.

Whilst training programmes have changed in recent years, the underlying experiences of many educators and students have not been substantially altered. The medical curriculum has come under particular criticisms for being overcrowded and relying too much on memorising facts.

- A shared vision for health education in the 21st century must now be developed. A major review of the content of the education system across undergraduate, graduate and continuing education for medical, nursing and other practitioners' training programmes must be initiated, to ensure the future health workforce is able to deliver all elements of patient-centred care.

Inter-professional training

The ability of health practitioners to work together collaboratively is critical to delivering patient-centred care. Common learning is due to be established in all pre-registration programmes in Higher Education institutions in England by 2004. However, a number of problems will need to be addressed for this to be achieved.

- Inter-professional training is likely to require a shift in focus towards more training being delivered in practice. Workforce Development Confederations must work with universities to develop appropriate work-based learning. A fair system of incentives and reward for staff who support work-based learning should be introduced.

- A key barrier to inter-professional training is the lack of evidence about its effectiveness. More investment in evaluating inter-professional learning must be provided in future.

Changing role models

A large part of medical training, particularly post-graduate training, is based around apprenticeship. Role models play a hugely important role in shaping the working practices, cultures and attitudes of staff.

- Role models and mentors need not necessarily be sought from within the same profession. Opportunities for doctors in training to learn from other practitioners, such as nurses and allied health professionals, should be explored in future.

● Revalidation should be developed beyond ensuring minimum standards so that is becomes a tool to help change the skills, attitudes and perceptions of existing practitioners within the NHS.

A new focus on support staff

The needs of the non-professionally qualified workforce have not been given sufficient priority to date and the lack of training support for this group of staff is a particular cause for concern.

● There are currently very few in service, part-time, work based courses open to the non-professionally qualified workforce. The NHSU should make the expansion of these courses a priority in future.

Making the skills escalator a reality

The development of a 'skills escalator' within the NHS, and its links to a reformed system of pay for non-medical staff through *Agenda for Change*, is hugely welcome. However, the lack of a common language or competence for vocational and professional occupations makes the transition from support worker to professional (or from 'porter to doctor') more difficult than it need be.

The use of occupational standards in professional areas like public health and social work are cited as evidence that it may be possible to base professional health qualifications on National Occupational Standards. However NOSs would have to be reformed to remove the arcane language and perceived bureaucracy of the awarding bodies, which have been a major cause of health professionals' resistance to using NOSs to date.

● Finding different points of entry into the professions and 'crediting in' people who have relevant experience could help support practitioners who wish to change career direction and improve relationships between different professional groups. The NHSU should explore the potential for a national Credit Accumulation and Transfer Scheme, to work across the health and social care sectors.

New health practitioners

There has been a tendency to presume that reforming working practices primarily involves 'delegating' doctors' responsibilities to nurses. New roles and responsibilities for other members of the health team must be explored in future, particularly in primary care and across the primary and secondary care sectors.

- For example, pharmacists could become responsible for managing the medicines of patients with long-term conditions, monitoring patients' health status and screening for previously undiagnosed conditions. Expanding pharmacists' responsibilities may require the current role of pharmacist to be split in two: creating a consultant pharmacist (responsible for medicines management and monitoring and screening patients) and a pharmacy technician (responsible for routine dispensing).

New types of practitioners who work across traditional professional divides and who focus on restoring health and wellbeing as well as treating ill health, may also need to emerge to improve patient outcomes.

- For example, Health Care Practitioners (who combine the skills of nurses, allied health professionals and doctors in training) are being piloted at Kingston Hospital. HCPs should now be explored in other settings particularly primary care and across the health and social care divide.

Creating a culture of innovation

A culture of innovation must be created in the NHS so that local providers are encouraged to explore new roles and responsibilities for staff and develop new types of practitioners.

The Government's role in this process must be to identify and remove any barriers to change, rather than attempt to impose new types of practitioners from the centre. The Government must end the perception, created by its pledges for more doctors and nurses, that its goal is to deliver 'more of the same'.

Creating a culture of innovation will also mean tackling the permission culture in the NHS. Local NHS Trusts often feel they cannot be innovative without securing prior permission, either from their Strategic Health

Authority or the Department of Health. So whilst staff are trained to take on new roles, they may be unable to put their skills into practice because their employing organisation is unable or unwilling to work in new ways.

The Government should work with professional organisations to identify and remove barriers to reform, such as the way staff are paid or unnecessary legal restrictions on working practices. However, cultural barriers are often as important as practical and legal obstructions in hindering the process of reform. Professional organisations have a key role to play in tackling this problem.

- Regulatory bodies must provide greater clarity about competencies, training and quality assurance for new roles as and when they develop.

- The Royal Colleges should publicise evidence about emerging roles and inform members who are interested in developing new ways of working where any legal barriers to change exist and when the barriers are more about custom and practice.

The future of regulation

Self-regulation has traditionally enshrined the assumption that only members of one's own profession are able to make a judgement on professional conduct. Regulatory bodies have already acknowledged the need to open up their internal working processes to patients, the public and other members of the health team. However, further changes will be necessary in future.

- Since professionals have to work in partnership with each other, as well as with patients, a standard of good practice which covers all professionals should be developed. This is something the new Council for the Regulation of Healthcare Professionals could be responsible for drawing up.

- The Council should also be empowered to manage a framework of regulation that can accommodate new practitioners who work across traditional professional divides, including the boundaries between health and social care.

- Another option would be to license or certify teams of practitioners, in addition to individual ones. For example, a diabetes patient could go to a diabetes care team that has been certified to ensure it provides a specific range and set of competencies.

- The potential for the revalidation process to help change the working practices, cultures and attitudes of existing staff has yet to be fully explored and is a key challenge facing regulatory bodies.

- The Government must consider, as a matter of urgency, the different options for regulating non-professionally qualified staff like healthcare assistants, particularly since their roles are likely to increase in future.

An inclusive and fair system of pay

Health workers' pay has traditionally been negotiated nationally though a process of annual appeals by organisations representing each of the different occupational groups. Some significant changes to this process have been made in recent years, such as the development of a job evaluation framework to form the basis of pay negotiations for non-medical staff through *Agenda for Change*.

However, doctors have not been part of this process. This could lead to problems in establishing a fair system of pay for nurses who have already taken on roles traditionally conducted by doctors, as well as for any attempt to further expand roles in the future.

- The separate negotiation of doctors' terms and conditions, and the disconnection from the pay scales of other professions should be reviewed in future.

- Over the longer term, disparities in pay between those working in health and social care will need to be addressed in order to facilitate the development of new roles and new practitioners who work across traditional health and social care divides.

Improving workforce planning

Whilst the introduction of Workforce Development Confederations has led to some improvements, workforce planning in the NHS is still based on the process of identifying gaps in the number of existing practitioners, rather than on assessing what types of practitioners with which sorts of skills are necessary to meet the needs of the local population. Universities' contracts with the NHS can serve to perpetuate the trend of delivering 'more of the same'.

- Workforce planning must shift from determining the supply of staff in specific disciplines who continue to perform the same tasks using the same methods toward assessing the adequacy of supply based on local population needs and likely future trends.

- A key issue is the need to ensure genuine integration of health and social care workforce planning and funding. Integrated workforce planning in selected areas should now be piloted.

System wide changes

The Government has recognised the need to devolve power and control within the health service. A more decentralised system could help tackle the 'permission culture' in the NHS and encourage more innovative approaches to workforce reform.

Proposals to introduce Foundation Trusts raise a series of difficult challenges that require careful attention, such as the need to establish an appropriate balance between national standards and local control, and the importance of ensuring an effective and coherent framework of local accountability. However, the potential advantages of community owned organisations like Foundation Trusts, particularly the role they might play in developing a greater sense of public and professional ownership over the management of services, and their ability to create a culture of innovation at the local level, suggests they should play an important role over the coming years.

1. Introduction

A challenge for progressive politics

NHS staff work for a public service that plays a critical role in delivering social justice. The NHS was created to ensure that those who need care receive it, regardless of their ability to pay. It embodies the recognition that an entitlement to key services like healthcare is a vital pre-condition for individual fulfilment and social citizenship.

More than fifty years later, opinion polls show consistently high levels of support for the NHS's founding principles and the staff who work in it. Yet during the intervening years, the important contribution made by the NHS and its workforce has not always been well reflected in practice. Levels of spending have consistently lagged behind health services in other European countries. The UK employs a lower proportion of staff in relation to the population than most other western healthcare systems. The pay and conditions of some members of the workforce have not fared well when compared to many private sector occupations, contributing to recruitment and retention difficulties. The result is that too many staff have to struggle to provide care in difficult and challenging circumstances.

The pressures facing the health workforce are set to increase in future. We are experiencing significant shifts in the nature and structure of society and a period of rapid technological advance. Patients are more informed and demanding. Only seven per cent of people who were born when the NHS was first established went to university. Now, 43 per cent of 18 to 30 year olds have had a university experience. People access health information from an increasingly wide range of sources, as evidenced by the explosion of lifestyle magazines and health websites. A decline in deference means traditional sources of authority – from the monarchy to politicians and clinicians – are questioned in ways unimaginable twenty years ago. New technologies are helping to transform the way many services are provided. Banks and supermarkets now offer 24-hour online access where services were once only available during the 9 to 5 working day. Scientific advances are expanding our knowledge about the causes and pathways of disease. Each day, discoveries from the human genome project herald the possibility of more personalised drugs and treatments, holding out the prospect of a major shift towards prevention or even genetic 'cure'. NHS staff have not been immune to these developments. Their working practices, attitudes and cultures have undergone substantial changes in recent years. New services are being developed to widen access to healthcare through the NHS Direct telephone advice line and new walk-in centres. Practitioners are starting to be trained to communicate better with patients and to provide more and better quality information. Professional regulatory bodies have recognised the need to open their doors to greater public scrutiny and now include 'lay' members on their boards. Many doctors have acknowledged they are no longer the sole custodians of power or knowledge within the NHS. Professional codes of conduct now promote the value of team-working and members of staff are taking new roles and responsibilities where old professional boundaries once held sway.

Yet despite these efforts, there is still much further to travel before the health workforce is ready to meet the demands of a 21st century healthcare system. Too many clinicians still fail to share information and control with patients, treating them as passive recipients rather than equal partners in their own treatment and care. Professional organisations and trades unions often remain pre-occupied with protecting their members' interests and identities, rather than with promoting the patient's interest or working with other members of the healthcare team. Restrictive practices and entrenched professional hierarchies can still work against the development of sufficiently flexible and responsive services. The weight of this hierarchy falls most heavily on the non-professionally qualified workforce,[1] which carries out many tasks that are vital to patient care but is often invisible in the process.

Reforming the health workforce therefore presents major challenges for Progressive politics. The invaluable contribution NHS staff make to delivering a more socially just society must be better recognised, and efforts to encourage people to enter the health professions redoubled, whilst simultaneously questioning whether these same professions require fundamental reform. Unnecessary demarcations between different occupational groups, which may hinder the provision of effective care, must be removed whilst at the same time continuing to address the system-wide barriers to change. Professional hierarchies and working practices which prevent the delivery of patient-centred care must be tackled, without belittling the commitment and sacrifices made by those same professions every day of their working lives.

The need to act

The NHS employs 1.25 million people in the UK, and estimates suggest that the social care sector employs a similar number. Between them, health and social care services employ one in ten of the UK working population. Staff costs account for around two thirds of all NHS expenditure. As Derek Wanless's interim report for the Treasury on the future health service argues:

> The number and mix of staff in the health service is a major determinant of the volume and quality of care... A health service without the right number of people, with the right skills, in the right locations will not deliver a high quality, comprehensive service to patients over the next two decades (Wanless 2001).

Whilst successive governments have talked about the need to give priority to reforming working practices, their overwhelming focus has been on structural change. Thus whilst the last Conservative Government called for reforms to the 'skills mix' of staff, the defining feature of its agenda was the attempt to introduce an internal market in the NHS by creating independent hospital Trusts and GP Fundholding. Likewise, the current Government made much of its desire to 'break down professional barriers' and 'tackle unnecessary demarcations' in the workforce when it was first elected. However, the past five years have been primarily characterised by structural change: the removal of GP Fundholding, the introduction of Primary Care Trusts, the abolition of health authorities and, most recently, the proposed creation of Foundation Hospitals.

There are a number of reasons why governments tend to focus on reforming the structures of the NHS rather than the working practices of those within it. Firstly, governments have often assumed that structural reforms are the key to improving health outcomes. Yet evidence on this issue is hard to come by (McCoy 2000; Wistow 2002). It is certainly clear that many practitioners regard structural change as irrelevant to their daily work. Recent research found only 20.8 per cent of staff are aware of any major structural changes that have occurred in the NHS since 1997. Those that are regard them as having little, if any relevance for the way in which they provide care (Curley *et al* 2003). Secondly, governments need to show progress within the course of an electoral cycle and educating the health workforce is a time consuming process. It takes twelve to thirteen years to train a consultant, far less to remove or create a new NHS structure.

The third reason for government preoccupation with structural reform is that past attempts to change working practices have proved notoriously difficult and controversial. Tensions between the medical profession and the state have been particularly problematic and began well before the inception of the NHS. Sir George Newman, the first Chief Medical Officer of the Ministry of Health, spoke to the BMA shortly after the Ministry's creation in 1920 and summarised the sentiments on either side:

> The state has seen in the profession a body insistent upon the privacy and individuality of its work, the sanctity of its traditions and the freedom of its engagements. The profession has seen in the state an organisation apparently devoted to the infringement of these traditions and incapable of putting anything worthy in their place. It has feared the imposition of some cast-iron system which might in practice make the practitioner of medicine servile, dependent and fettered (quoted Rivett 1998).

The medical profession's resistance to the Labour Government's plans to nationalise health services after the second world war has been well documented. The fear of political interference in clinical practice led to an implicit bargain being struck between the state and the profession (Klein 1983). The terms of the agreement effectively meant that the Government would set the overall level of funding for the NHS whilst the profession would be free to control the way the money was spent, with doctors deciding on the priority for treating patients within the available resources. There was a degree of collusion between the Government and the medical profession about not interfering in each other's sphere of responsibility (Alberti and Ham 2002).

However, since this bargain was struck, doctors have perceived an increasing encroachment on their professional autonomy by politicians, particularly through their proxy at the local level, the health service manager. This was one of the main factors behind the rejection of the consultant contract in England and Wales (Smith 2002). It has been reported that the Chief Medical Officer for England, Professor Sir Liam Donaldson, was told by a senior consultant that the contract's rejection was 'payback time for the Griffiths report[2]' (Lyall 2003). Organisations representing health professionals now frequently complain about the number of targets being set by central government, which local managers are required to deliver. The Chairman of the British Medical Association Dr Ian Bogle has complained:

> we now have a healthcare system driven...by spreadsheets and tick boxes. An NHS underpinned by production-line values in pushing doctors into becoming a bunch of technicians at the beck and call of ministers and managers, whose worth is measured in terms of output and nothing else.

A sense of disengagement with the process of reform now exists in many quarters. Clinicians feel they have to deliver patient care 'at the front line' and deal with the consequences if things go wrong, or if patients get angry and complain. Yet at the same time, they feel they are not given a sufficient say in how the NHS's priorities are set or where the extra money coming into the service is being spent. There is a profound contrast between the responsibility staff feel for providing patient care, and the degree of power and influence they feel they are able to exert over 'the system'. Addressing this problem is one of the most important issues facing the NHS and will be critical to the success of future workforce reforms.

The lack of a coherent vision

Professional organisations, trades unions and Government all agree that further changes to working practices will be required in the years ahead. Yet there is little agreement about what the overall shape of the future health workforce should look like. The British Medical Association (BMA) has called for a hugely expanded role for nurses. It suggests that nurses will replace doctors as the first 'port of call' in primary care with clinical nurse specialists co-ordinating the movement of patients across the system (British Medical Association 2002). The BMA does not, however, envisage non-professionally qualified workers taking on more responsibility as nurses roles expand, something the Wanless report regards as critical if nurses are to help reduce doctors' workloads. An extra 70,000 Health Care Assistants (in addition to the projected increase in demand of 74,000) may be needed if nurses are to take on substantially enhanced roles in future (Wanless 2002).

The Royal College of Physicians (RCP) has put forward a somewhat different solution. It suggests that the problems being faced by physicians are unlikely to be solved by training existing health care professionals to take over some of the duties of medical staff. It instead proposes the development of a new type of healthcare practitioner – the physicians assistant: a semi-autonomous professional who carries out similar tasks to physicians including examinations, diagnosis, treatment (including referral) and prescribing. The RCP suggests the BMA's model is neither possible (due to the shortage of properly trained nurses), nor desirable, since it would take nurses away from other important clinical areas and fail to deliver cost-effective care (Royal College of Physicians 2001).

These different visions for the future are perhaps unsurprising. The primary purpose of professional organisations and trades unions is to protect and promote the interests of their members, rather than those of other practitioners or, more importantly, patients. Thus, whilst initiatives which seek to reduce doctors' workloads by expanding nurses roles can help to improve both doctors working lives and the quality of patient care (for example by reducing waiting times), if nurses are also in short supply and become overburdened, the implications – for nurses and patients – are less clear.

Assessing whether changes in working practices deliver genuine improvements in patient care is not straightforward. For example, the professionalisation of nursing has arguably helped improve the quality of care by challenging unnecessary inflexibilities in doctors' working practices, and improving nurses recruitment and retention rates through increased status and better career progression. However, this same professionalisation may have also led to the entrenchment of occupational hierarchies between nurses and other members of the workforce, such as health care assistants, which may not be in the patient's interest. The increasing specialisation of the health workforce is another case in point. Whilst specialisation can help improve the quality of care as knowledge and expertise becomes concentrated in the hands of a few practitioners, it can also lead to fragmentation or duplications in the process of care and the devaluation of generalist skills.

Unspoken differences in professional culture and attitude can undermine a shared sense about what is really in the patients' best interest. There are often deeply held views about the specific contribution different practitioners make to the process of care, which are in turn closely related to the practitioner's personal as well as professional identity. These views are difficult to quantify and rarely discussed openly, but they nevertheless exert a powerful influence on staff relations and the way in which care is provided. Two anecdotes serve to illustrate this point. In response to a presentation about patients' desire for greater involvement and information at a government sponsored conference about the future of the NHS, the senior medic chairing the event commented that whilst patients might want their doctor to talk to them more, what was really important was that the doctor knew how to carry out the operation. A senior Government nurse called for the 'future proofing' of nursing during a meeting at a major nursing conference, and her fellow panel member suggested this meant clearly defining that the essence of nursing 'was love'.[3]

These stories show how professionals can identify themselves with very different responsibilities or attributes in the process of care, when in reality these skills and qualities should be, and indeed are, shared. A study of medical and nursing cultures has suggested that there are in fact no distinguishable differences between the 'core values' that underpin both professions. However, their different cultures and histories lead to alternative interpretations as to how these values might be pursued in practice (National Primary Care Research and Development Centre 1997).

Defining patient-centred care

The objective of any reform of the health workforce must be to improve the quality of care being provided so that it better meets the needs of patients. This requires a clear and shared definition about what constitutes high quality, patient-centred care.

It has already been suggested that professional organisations and trades unions can conflate their members' interests with those of the patient, when this may not necessarily be the case. The Government has also failed to develop a persuasive definition of patient centred care, despite its claim that 'Our vision is a health service designed around the patient' (Department of Health 2000a). The Government sees patient-centred care as primarily about making access to services more timely and convenient and improving patients choices about where and when their operations take place. Whilst these are certainly important features of a patient-centred system, they do not amount to a sufficiently broad or coherent definition. A comprehensive definition of patient-centred care would, for example, recognise the need to prevent people from becoming ill, and to promote and restore health and wellbeing. A definition of patient-centred care based on an awareness of likely future trends would recognise that the care needs of people with chronic conditions, who will form the majority of service users in future, are not based on having infrequent and intense periods of care such as hospital operations but on receiving regular, low levels of care in their local community and within their home.

In order to shape a vision for the future health workforce, we need to develop a shared definition of what high quality, patient-centred care is and a shared understanding of how the workforce might need to change in order to deliver this goal. This is what *The Future Health Worker* seeks to provide.

2. Patient-centred care: towards a definition

The term 'patient-centred care' has been used to indicate both an approach to organising health services and working practices, and a particular style of interaction between patients and practitioners. The concept of re-organising health services around the needs of patients first emerged in the US in the 1980s when hospitals were attempting to meet increasing patient demand within a difficult financial climate (Greene 1994). A group of management consultants who had been improving manufacturing processes claimed their techniques could equally be applied to the acute health care sector. It was claimed that providing better services to patients could be achieved at the same time as meeting the financial 'bottom line' by reconfiguring services around patients' needs rather than around traditional professional or institutional priorities (Lathrop 1993).

The Conservative Government adopted a similar approach in the UK during the early 1990s when it attempted to introduce market principles to the NHS. *The NHS and Community Care Act* (1990) created NHS Trusts: supposedly autonomous institutions that were intended to compete with one another to secure contracts from Health Authorities and GP Fundholders. It was hoped this would lead to hospitals reconfiguring their services to provide more patient-centred care. The creation of NHS Trusts, alongside the introduction of general management into the health system, was also intended to tackle professional tribalism and encourage greater collaboration and corporate identity amongst the NHS workforce.

During the 1990s, managers were keen to emphasise that the purpose of reconfiguring services 'around the needs of patients' was to improve the quality of care being provided rather than to improve cost-efficiency alone. However, the pressure on Trusts to reduce their costs in the new competitive environment at a time of constrained funding after 1992-3 was certainly an important motivating factor (NHSE 1996). The Conservative Government consistently blurred the goals of improving patient care and lowering staff costs, particularly in its approach to reforming the working practices of staff (Department of Health and Social Security 1986). This led to criticisms that the real objective of 'patient-centred care' was cost-cutting through the 'dilution' of the professions, particularly nursing – a concern that grew when the numbers of qualified staff were substantially reduced between 1991 and 1992.

The Conservative Government's health policy was anathema to many NHS staff. Attempts to introduce a market-ethos into the NHS were criticised for increasing inequalities in access to services by prioritising GP Fundholders' patients over patients of non-Fundholding GPs, for promoting competition over collaboration, and for reducing the quality of care by putting cost-cutting before clinical effectiveness. The association of the term 'patient-centred care' with these policies means some sections of the workforce fear renewed interest in the concept from today's Government implies a return to a 1990s agenda. Such perceptions are re-enforced by the striking similarities between the policies pursued by the previous Government and the current one. Some ministers may be reluctant to use the language of the market, yet the introduction of independent Foundation Hospitals, the emphasis on promoting patient choice, and the expansion of the private sectors role in the provision of care has led commentators to conclude 'we are undoubtedly seeing the development of a regulated internal market in healthcare' (Le Grand 2003).

However, the term 'patient-centred care' has also been linked with recent research into the nature of individual patient's interactions with health practitioners. Qualitative research has explored what users want from their services and what makes care 'patient-centred'. Definitions of quality from both health and social care users consistently emphasise the nature of their relationship with practitioners, in addition to material aspects such as how quickly patients receive care or the quality of facilities (Williams and Calnan 1991; Walker *et al* 1998; Turner 2000; Henwood 2001; Kendall 2001).

There have been extensive studies investigating patient-centredness in doctors' interactions with patients. Doctors who work to the patients' agenda, who listen and respond to what the patients say, who provide patients with high quality, relevant information and who develop relationships which treat patients as partners in the process of care are said to use a 'patient-centred' approach. This contrasts with what has been termed a 'disease-centred' style, where the doctor specifically leads communication and seeks to diagnose the patient's problem through text book style enquiries about the patient's symptoms and medical history. Higher degrees of patient-centredness in doctors' styles have been clearly related to higher patient satisfaction rates (Williams and Calnan 1991).

Others suggest that patient-centred care is about much more than how practitioners communicate with patients during consultations, although this is certainly an integral feature.

Box 2.1 Patient-Centred Care for hospital inpatients
(Gerteis *et al* 1993)

● Respect for patients' values, preferences, and expressed needs (including impact of illness and treatment on quality of life, involvement in decision-making, dignity and autonomy)

● Coordination and integration of care (including clinical care, ancillary and support services and 'front-line' care);

● Information, communication, and education (including clinical status, progress and prognosis, processes of care, facilitation of autonomy, self-care and health promotion);

● Physical comfort (including pain management, help with activities of daily living, surroundings and hospital environment);

● Emotional support and alleviation of fear and anxiety (including clinical status, treatment and prognosis, impact of illness on self and family, financial impact of illness);

● Involvement of family and friends (including social and emotional support, involvement in decision-making, support for care-giving, impact on family dynamics and functioning);

● Transition and continuity (including information about medication and danger signals to look out for after leaving hospital, co-ordination and discharge planning, clinical, social, physical and financial support).

Qualitative research by Gerteis *et al* (1993) identifies a number of features that are critical to patient-centred care. Patient centred care shows respect for patients' preferences and expressed needs, giving patients abundant opportunities to be informed and involved in decision making but understands that patients' preferences are likely to change over time and to depend on the clinical problems in question. Patient-centred care effectively co-ordinates services within the healthcare system and outside it, managing smooth transitions from one setting to another, or from a health care to a self-care setting. Genuinely patient centred care is based on a broad understanding of patients' needs, recognising that suffering is about more than just physical pain and other distressing symptoms and includes a significant emotional dimension. Patient-centred care sees individual patient's needs in the context of their wider family and community resources and includes the family members and friends who are involved in the process of care, recognising their needs and contributions. It also provides high quality, tailored and responsive information and education to patients about their particular illness and treatment options, and about self-care and health promotion.

Box 2.2 Establishing Aims for the 21st Century Health Care System (Institute of Medicine 2001)

- *Safe* – avoiding injuries to patients from the care that is intended to help them
- *Effective* – providing services based on scientific knowledge to all who could benefit and refraining from providing services to those not likely to benefit (avoiding under-use and overuse, respectively)
- *Patient-centred* – providing care that is respectful of and responsive to individual patient preferences, needs, and values and ensuring that patients values guide all clinical decisions
- *Timely* – reducing waits and sometimes harmful delays for both those who receive and those who give care
- *Efficient* – avoiding waste, including waste of equipment, supplies, ideas and energy
- *Equitable* – providing care that does not vary in quality because of personal characteristics such as gender, ethnicity, geographic location, and socio-economic status

---

The influential work of the US Institute of Medicine's 'Quality of Health Care in America' project identifies patient-centred care as one of the six key dimensions around which improvements in health services will need to be made in order to better meet the needs of patients. Whilst patient-centred care is identified as a separate element, the Institute recognises that their six quality dimensions are in fact closely related. For example, in order to be responsive to individual patients, care must also be timely so that unnecessary delays in treatment are removed. Ensuring healthcare is effective (based on the best available scientific knowledge about which interventions would benefit the individual patient) helps ensure it is also equitable, in other words that it does not vary on account of factors such as geographic location or socio-economic status.

IPPR's definition

The definition of patient-centred care used in this report builds on the different analyses outlined above. Our definition is based on an understanding of what patients want from their health services, but also on the evidence of what is necessary to deliver better patient outcomes.

It provides a framework for improving current services but also seeks to anticipate likely future trends.

High quality, patient-centred care can be summarised by five broad characteristics:

- *Safe and effective.* Patients should not be harmed by the care that is intended to help them. Care which is unsafe can not only harm individual patients but also make the overall health system less cost-effective. Patients should receive care which is based on the best available evidence to determine whether an intervention produces better outcomes than the alternatives. Evidence-based practice requires that those who give care consistently avoid both under use of effective care and overuse of ineffective care (Institute of Medicine 2001).

- *Promoting health and wellbeing.* Genuinely patient-centred care not only effectively treats illness but also seeks to prevent ill health and promote good health (Stewart 2001). Preventing people from becoming ill so they do not have to go to hospital for more invasive and potentially dangerous procedures; rehabilitating older people so that they can live independently rather than remaining in hospital or in a care home – these goals are important because they are likely to improve patient satisfaction, lead to better health outcomes, and improve the overall cost-effectiveness of the system (Wanless 2002). Promoting health and wellbeing has been an under-explored feature of patient-centred care to date.

- *Integrated and seamless.* Patient-centred care effectively co-ordinates services within the NHS and between the NHS and other sectors, for example social care. Integrated services take a 'whole person' approach, seeking to meet users' social and emotional needs, as well as their physical and medical ones. Integrated services recognise that an individual's needs are related to those of their family and wider community and therefore seek to take action at all these levels. Care which is based on an understanding of the holistic nature of people's needs is a key priority from the users' perspective. Research suggests it is also critical to improving outcomes (Wistow 2002).

●   *Informing and empowering.* Providing patients with high quality information, and enabling those who want to to become equal partners in decisions is a key feature of patient-centred care. IPPR has previously argued that patient empowerment must go beyond simply informing and involving patients to supporting them to take on appropriate responsibilities (Kendall 2001). There is a growing body of evidence that enabling patients to share responsibility for their wellbeing and care can lead to better health outcomes, and help reduce inappropriate use of services (Cooper 2001a).

●   *Timely and convenient.* A top priority for patients is that services are delivered in a timely and responsive manner. Timely services also play an important role in improving health outcomes and ensuring the overall cost-effectiveness of system: if access to healthcare is inappropriately delayed and a patient's condition worsens, or if patients end up in Accident and Emergency departments because they cannot access services in primary care, then care may be both less clinically and cost-effective (Wanless 2002).

The following chapter explores each of these five characteristics in greater detail. It analyses the contribution that health practitioners make to achieving these characteristics (including how this contribution may be shaped by the wider health system) and the degree to which they are important objectives of current workforce reforms.

3. Patient-centred care: the contribution of the workforce

Safe and effective

A fundamental feature of patient-centred care is that it is safe. Patients should not be harmed by the care that is intended to help them and the healthcare environment should be safe for all patients in all of its process all of the time (Institute of Medicine 2000). Patient-centred care is also effective. Effective care is based on the use of systematically acquired evidence to determine whether an intervention produces better outcomes than the alternatives. Evidence-based practice requires that those who give care consistently avoid both under-use of effective care and over-use of ineffective care (Institute of Medicine 2001).

Safe and effective health care is crucial to improving outcomes for patients and ensuring the overall cost-effectiveness of the health system. It is also integral to building trust in health practitioners and the NHS as a whole. The issue of trust is particularly important in healthcare: although patients are becoming increasingly informed, there are still major asymmetries of information between the users and providers of care. In recent years, the safety and effectiveness of health services in general – and trust in health professionals in particular – have been brought into question by a series of incidents of negligent and even criminal practice in the NHS.[1]

Serious failures in practice are uncommon relative to the high volume of care that is provided, and criminal behaviour is even more rare. There is nevertheless worrying evidence about the rates of serious medical failures in the NHS. Best research estimates suggest that each year, adverse events in which harm is caused to patients occur in around 10 per cent of admissions, or at a rate in excess of 850,000. Around 400 people die or are seriously injured in adverse events involving medical devices. Nearly 10,000 people are reported to have experienced serious adverse reactions to drugs. These events are estimated to cost £2 billion a year in additional hospital stays alone, without taking into account any of the human or wider economic costs. Hospital acquired infections, around 15 per cent of which may be avoidable, are estimated to cost the NHS nearly £1 billion a year (Department of Health 2000b).

The UK is not alone in facing this problem: it has been estimated that between 44,000 and 98,000 Americans die each year from medical errors which could be prevented (Institute of Medicine 2000). Research also raises serious questions about the effectiveness of a substantial proportion of healthcare. The now infamous claim that only 20 to 25 per cent of medical decisions are 'evidence-based' first emerged during the 1970s. When Kerr White suggested to his fellow epidemiologist Archie Cochrane (after whom the Cochrane Collaboration is named) that only fifteen to twenty per cent of physicians' interventions were supported by objective evidence that they did more good than harm, his colleague replied: 'Kerr, you're a damned liar! You know it isn't more than ten per cent.'[5] Shortly after (1978), the US Congress's Office of Technology Assessment reported that 'only ten to twenty per cent of all procedures currently used in medical practice have been shown to be efficacious by controlled trial' (a charge it repeated in the early 1980s). Since then, numerous academics and practitioners have argued that evidence other than that provided by controlled trials must be taken into account when assessing the effectiveness of healthcare interventions. Taking this approach, recent research suggests that 82 per cent of interventions in general medicine (Ellis *et al* 1995) and 81 per cent of interventions in general practice (Gill *et al* 1996) are evidence-based.

The Institute of Medicine argues: 'It is clearly not possible to base all care on sound scientific evidence and certainly not exclusively on randomised controlled trials, which narrowly define study populations and exclude or control for factors that are inevitably relevant in real world healthcare settings.' However, this still means scant or no evidence of either effectiveness or ineffectiveness exists for a substantial proportion of health care interventions (Institute of Medicine 2001). Studies indicate this problem is experienced across primary, secondary and tertiary care in all western industrialised countries (Booth 2000).

Barriers to safe and effective care

Professional values, cultures and working practices have had an important effect on the safety and effectiveness of healthcare. In a recent speech the ex-President of the General Medical Council, Sir Donald Irvine, explored the reasons behind the poor practice of doctors like

Rodney Ledward, Richard Neale and others. He argued that whilst such cases are undoubtedly extreme examples, their root cause lies in key characteristics of the medical culture such as the ingrained sanctity of clinical autonomy:

> We have tended to resent criticisms of clinical care, to be too tolerant of poor practice and resistant to openness about professional performance. We have insisted on our own take on basics like accountability, consent and communication with patients. Of course there are other systemic causes which together constitute a general systems failure. But healthcare clinical systems are built and operated by people, prominent amongst whom are doctors (Irvine 2002).

The final report of the Bristol Royal Infirmary Inquiry also illustrated how a monopoly of medical power can lead to disastrous consequences. The report showed that a 'club culture' and an imbalance of power between medical and other members of staff were major factors behind the poor quality of care provided to children in Bristol. These contributed to a lack of teamwork and the failure of staff to communicate and work together effectively in the interests of patients. However, the Inquiry emphasised that flaws in the way the wider healthcare system is organised also played a major role, highlighting issues such as the absence of systematic mechanisms for monitoring the clinical performance of professionals or hospitals (Kennedy *et al* 2001).

Professional attitudes can also influence attempts to encourage more widespread use of evidence-based care. For example, one of the main reasons given for the substantial variations in the proportion of day care surgery carried out by NHS Trusts is that clinicians do not accept some procedures are suitable for day surgery, even though they are considered so by leading clinicians in the field (Audit Commission 2001). Some doctors believe evidence-based practice implies a rigid and even mindless adherence to evidence drawn from randomised controlled trials. However, leading advocates – who include many doctors – argue that true evidence-based practice is about combining the best available clinical evidence from systematic research with individual clinical expertise. External clinical evidence can inform but never replace individual clinical experience, not least because patients' choices must also be taken into account in the process of effective care.

It is important to recognise there are also important system-wide barriers to practitioners delivering evidence-based care. There is a plethora of journals and peer-reviewed papers on the emerging evidence base. It has been estimated that doctors would need to read 19 articles a day, 365 days a year to keep up to speed with 'evidence-based' practice (Davidoff et al 1995). However, most practising clinicians have very little time to acquaint themselves with even a small proportion of this information. Finding ways of addressing this problem, for example through effective use of information technology, is a major challenge facing all healthcare systems.

Recent changes

A range of initiatives is being implemented to ensure individual practitioners, and the NHS as a whole, deliver safer, more effective patient care. The Chief Medical Officer's report *An Organisation with a Memory*, acknowledged that one of the biggest challenges in moving towards a safer health system is changing the culture of blame (Department of Health 2000b), something the final report of the Bristol Royal Infirmary Inquiry also emphasised (Kennedy et al 2001). Both reports suggest that instead of treating errors as personal failures, they should be used as opportunities to improve the system and prevent future harm. The Government's response has been to establish a mandatory, national reporting scheme for adverse health care events and near misses in the NHS, alongside a new independent body, the National Patient Safety Agency (Department of Health 2001a). These initiatives build on the lessons learnt about how to improve safety in other sectors, such as aviation, and other countries like the US (Institute of Medicine 2000).

A key theme in the report of the Bristol Royal Infirmary Inquiry is the need to break down barriers between professionals in order to address imbalances in power between medics and other members of staff. The report calls for inter-professional training to be encouraged to ensure more open and effective team working, for the establishment of an overarching body to co-ordinate and align the activities of professional regulatory bodies and ensure they work to serve the patient's interest, and for compulsory Continuing Professional Development, appraisal and revalidation for health professionals to ensure skills and knowledge are kept up to date.

A number of initiatives had already been set in train to address these issues before the Bristol report was published, and additional proposals have also since emerged. A range of mechanisms are now being used to set and monitor standards across the NHS, including National Service Frameworks, the National Institute for Clinical Excellence and the Commission for Healthcare Audit and Inspection. 'Common learning' is due to be implemented in all pre-registration programmes in Higher Education institutions in England by 2004 (Department of Health 2001b). A Council for the Regulation of Healthcare Professionals is being established from April 2003 to strengthen and co-ordinate the system of professional self-regulation and the new General Social Care Council is registering key practitioners working in the field of social care. An Electronic Library for Health – a 'virtual' library providing access to information about health problems, their causes and treatment – is also being set up to support clinicians in adopting evidence based practice.

Changes to the internal workings of regulatory bodies that were already taking place were given added impetus by the Bristol report. Regulatory bodies have recognised the need become more open and transparent: the General Medical Council (GMC), for example, has increased the proportion of its members from the public from 12 to 40 per cent. The GMC has also set out an explicit statement of professional values and standards in *Good Medical Practice* and in 1998, the concept of medical professionalism was extended to embrace the clinical team. New doctors have to demonstrate they comply with these standards when they first join the register, and those already on the register will have to offer evidence of their continuing compliance in order to stay on it once very five years. A new process of appraisal has also been launched for both consultants (from April 2001) and GPs (from April 2002). The aim of appraisal is to help doctors consolidate and improve on good performance, although it may also help identify poor performance at an early stage. A new Code of Professional Conduct has also been introduced for nursing (Nursing and Midwifery Council 2002). The Code aims to inform nurses, other professionals, patients and employers of the standards of professional conduct required from nurses. It too emphasises that team working is critical, stating that the health team includes patients and their carers, as well as other practitioners.

Many of these developments are still at an early stage, and their impact will be hard to determine for some while. Future challenges to the delivery of safe and effective health care – such as the move towards more services provided in local communities rather than in acute hospitals – are also on the horizon.

Barriers to the successful implementation of existing policies have already emerged. For example, a number of issues have been raised in relation to inter professional training. These include the importance of building an evidence base about its effectiveness (Humphris and McLeod Clark 2002), practical issues such as the imbalance in student numbers in the different professions and the fact that not all medical nursing and other schools are located on the same site, and addressing concerns amongst some sections of the workforce that the real aim of inter professional training is to 'deconstruct' the professions and cut costs and jobs (Hale 2002).

There are other areas where workforce reforms will be necessary to ensure care is safer and more effective in future. Despite clear commitments to improving patient safety and standards, the increasing stringency seen in relation to continuing professional development, and a growing framework of monitoring and inspection, these measures have yet to have a direct impact on a major section of the health workforce: non-professionally qualified staff. In future, it will be anathema for key members of the health team to be entirely un-regulated as is currently the case for non-professionally qualified staff, particularly if their roles are increased. Whilst the Government has indicated its willingness to address this issue, no actual changes to the regulation of this section of the workforce have so far occurred (Rogers 2002; Johnson *et al* 2002).

Delivering safe and effective care has profound implications for the way future health workers are trained. Professionals will need to be able to identify errors and hazards in care; have the skills necessary to design processes of care and measure their effectiveness, even when the members of the team that care for a patient are not in the same physical locale; and understand how to find new knowledge as it continually expands, evaluate its significance and claims of effectiveness and decide how to incorporate it into practice. Clinical education does not currently prepare practitioners for these roles. As the Institute for Medicine argues (2001):

> The traditional emphasis in clinical education, particularly medical education, is on teaching a core of knowledge, much of it focused on the basic mechanisms of disease and pathophysiological principles. Given the expansiveness and dynamic nature of the science base in health care, this approach should be expanded to teach how to manage knowledge and use effective tools that can support clinical decision making.

Learning about evidence based practice requires an emphasis on teaching the application of critical appraisal skills in actual patient care settings and experience in conducting literature searches and applying methodological rules to the evaluation and understanding of evidence (Evidence-Based Medicine Working Group 1992). It also means changing traditional methods of continuing education. Formal conferences and dissemination of educational materials have been shown to have little effect by themselves on changing clinician behaviours or health outcomes (Davis *et al* 1995). The use of decision support tools may be necessary to provide strong incentives for clinicians to undertake continuing learning. Studies indicate that computer assisted diagnosis and management can improve quality (Durieux *et al* 2000; Evans *et al* 1998) and automated reminder systems can help improve compliance with clinical practice guidelines (Balas *et al* 2000; Shea *et al* 1996). New information technologies are therefore likely to play a key role in providing continuing education in future.

Promoting health and wellbeing

Academics and policy makers have long argued that the NHS is a service which seeks to treat ill health rather than prevent it from occurring in the first place. The policies and investment priorities of successive governments have focused on 'downstream' healthcare interventions, which usually take place in hospitals, rather than on 'upstream' activities to tackle the underlying determinants of health and promote health and wellbeing, which are traditionally conducted in the community (see for example Ashton and Seymour 1988; Appleby and Coote 2002).

The focus on healthcare, rather than health, means many people suffer from diseases which could be prevented. The major causes of mortality and morbidity in the 21st century will be cardiovascular disease, lung cancer, diabetes and other long term illnesses. These conditions are closely related to individual behaviour such as physical inactivity and excessive calorie, tobacco and alcohol consumption. For example, smoking accounts for more than 20 per cent of incidents of Coronary Heart Disease, and high cholesterol levels which are mainly due to diet account for 43 per cent. Lifestyle factors are in turn heavily influenced by socio-economic status: 35 per cent of men in manual groups smoke compared to 23 per cent in non-manual groups, and 25 per cent of children aged 2 to 15 years in affluent families eat fruit more than once a day, compared to just 15 per cent in poorer families (Wanless 2002).

The impact of these inequalities on the individuals involved, and the health system as a whole, is profound. People from the most disadvantaged groups in society die on average five years before their most advantaged counterparts. Research indicates that if all social classes were to match the incidences of limiting long standing illness found in social class 1, hospital admission rates would fall by 6 per cent (Wanless 2002). A lack of services which seek to prevent ill health and promote good health also result in many patients being trapped in acute care when they would better be cared for in the community or at home. Research suggests that as many as a third of people who occupy acute hospital beds have needs that are not commensurate with that level of care (Vaughan and Withers 2002). This is neither good for the patients who are unnecessarily trapped in hospital, nor for those patients who need access to acute care but cannot get it.

The current Government has acknowledged the existence of health inequalities and their close relationship with social and economic factors – in stark contrast to the previous Conservative government, which for many years denied such inequalities existed and only towards the end of its administration acknowledged the presence of some 'health variations'. A number of policies have been put in place to give greater emphasis to public health. One of the key tasks of Primary Care Trusts is improving the health of their local population. The initial decision to reject the use of national inequalities targets has now been reversed. Although early enthusiasm for local initiatives to tackle health inequalities such as Health Action Zones has cooled, the importance of linking efforts to improve health and wellbeing with wider programmes to regenerate local communities and tackle social exclusion, such as the New Deal for Communities and Sure Start, has been recognised. A number of programmes to tackle individual health behaviour, such as smoking cessation, are also being introduced.

However, the overwhelming focus of the current political and policy agenda is still on improving health services rather than on improving health. National health inequality targets do not have real 'bite' compared to key performance indicators such as targets to improve waiting times. Whilst Primary Care Trusts have been given a mandate to improve health, the enormity of the task they face in both commissioning and providing health services means public health will inevitably be a secondary concern (Naish 2002). The lack of priority given to public health in this country is also apparent from the lower levels of spending compared to other European countries. The UK invests around one per cent in public health as a proportion of total healthcare expenditure, compared to around three to five percent in Finland and the Netherlands (Lister 2002).

Shifting the focus of care towards prevention may be even more important in future. The health service is currently based upon a model of diagnose and cure. However, knowledge emerging from the exploration of the human genome is likely to provide opportunities for pre-symptomatic prediction and the prevention of disease through the use of genetic tests. These opportunities will not be confined to rare single gene disorders, such as Huntingdon's disease, but will apply to a host of more common conditions including cancer, asthma and Alzheimer's. Unless health services and practitioners are prepared for the changes the new genetics will bring, and given the right support and incentives to do so, important opportunities for preventing illness and improving health may be lost (Lenaghan 1998).

The medical model of health: a brief history of the professions

The reason why services have tended to focus on treating ill health, rather than promoting or restoring good health, are complex. It has been argued that the power and control afforded to doctors within the health system – and the subsequent dominance of the medical model of health – has been a major contributing factor, exerting a powerful influence on the way health practitioners work, how they relate to one another, and their relationships with patients and local communities (see for example Salvage 2002; Naish 2002).

A brief history of the medical profession helps illuminate this point. Medicine emerged as an organised profession in the 19th century. As Davies (1999) persuasively argues, Victorian attitudes to class and gender were central in shaping the structure of the health workforce and medicine's dominance of it, as well as the relationships between patients and professionals. Thus Florence Nightingale's decision to model professional nursing on the Victorian household accorded with the prevailing social order: the doctor/father at the head of the system issuing orders, the nurse/wife obediently carrying them out, and the patient/child gratefully and silently receiving care (Davies 1999).

The medical profession's definition of, and subsequent control of, its knowledge base and its ability to control entry into training were crucial ingredients in its success. These factors came to be seen as critical yardsticks by which other practitioners could justify their claims to be a profession. Occupations such as nursing were considered to have failed the test and were famously consigned to being 'semi -professions' because of their inferior knowledge base (Etzioni 1969). Nursing's initial struggle to gain acceptance as a profession has had a major influence on its later development and its relations with other practitioners such as healthcare assistants (Rogers 2002).

During the first half of the twentieth century, there was a shift away from care being delivered by a range of practitioners in local communities towards treatment being provided by professionals in institutions. Hospitals became the power base of medicine. By the time the NHS was established in 1948, consultants were so powerful that their mouths were famously 'stuffed with gold' in order to secure their agreement to the new institution. The power and status of those working in hospitals is still apparent today. As Harrison and Dixon argue (2000), medicine's rewards are greatest in areas of specialist care in hospitals but 'professional prizes glitter less obviously for the generalist, such as the geriatrician or general practitioner, for whom the emphasis of practice is to provide low intensity services at, or near, the patients' home and to keep patients out of hospital.'

The dominance of the medical model of health has also influenced the development of the public health workforce, with public health science – and public health doctors – largely dominating other contributions (Naish 2002).[6] Again, history helps shed some light on this issue. Until 1970, public health practitioners such as medical officers of health, health visitors and school nurses were employed by local authorities, not the NHS. However, the concern that public health lay on the margins of NHS activity, and therefore lacked power and status within it, led to public health being refashioned into a professional medical specialism, following the recommendations of the 1988 Acheson report.

Public health departments were created within the NHS. These were run by Directors of Public Health: public health doctors whose focus was on building the public health science base using the disciplines of epidemiology, health economics and medical statistics. Health visitors and other practitioners who had traditionally been regarded as public health workers, were moved into the NHS but located outside public health departments. This led both to the fracturing of the public health workforce and the separation of public health science from public health practice, namely 'hands-on' work with local communities (Naish 2002). Public health departments became involved in the process of commissioning health care (as opposed to commissioning for health) following the introduction of the purchaser provider split in the NHS in the late 1980s, something not all were enthusiastic about (Levenson 1997). However this role, combined with the establishment of a model of public health based primarily on public health science (and mandatory medical leadership), further isolated and separated the public health function and workforce (Naish 2002).

The 1990s and early 2000s have brought challenges to the dominance of public health medicine from public health managers and academics who undertake equivalent work to public health doctors without commensurate pay, status or career opportunities and government policy has supported this trend. For example, every Primary

Care Trust has to appoint a Director of Public Health, a post which is now open to non-medical appointees. The Chief Medical Officer's report on strengthening the public health function has also emphasised the importance of community development (Department of Health 2001). However, whilst opening up Director of Public Health posts to non-medics has been welcomed 'they have not yet sufficiently changed or challenged the hierarchy of public health in which the science based end of the continuum still dominates' (Naish 2002). Some commentators have called for a new generation of Public Health Leaders to drive forward the public health agenda in future. These leaders could have a community development background, be trained in environmental health or housing, or in health visiting or health promotion, as well as medicine. Their role would be to co-ordinate activities within local communities to deliver on public health objectives. This would require strong leadership skills and the ability to bring together practitioners with very diverse backgrounds (Tennant and Woodhead 2002).

The medical model of health: other contributory factors

It would be wrong to place the entire responsibility for the dominance of the medical model of health on the shoulders of the medical profession. The short-termism of our political system must also shoulder a degree of blame. Politicians are inevitably driven by the need to show results within the course of an electoral cycle, yet the benefits of upstream intervention to prevent ill health may not be seen for many years. The media also plays an important role. Greater prominence is given to stories of patients left waiting on trolleys in Accident and Emergency departments or to examples of miracle cures, than to research or initiatives which demonstrate prevention is better than cure.

Questions about the effectiveness of different public health interventions have been another important factor preventing a greater focus on public health. Gowman and Coote argue (2000) that public health evidence has too often been hard to come by, of questionable quality and uncertain relevance. This lack of evidence has lead to public health practitioners lacking confidence in their ability to make an impact and in the willingness of their colleagues to accept they have the ability to do so. However, Gowman and Coote also question the traditional hierarchy of evidence (a subject this report has already referred to) where evidence from Randomised Controlled Trials is considered the best and most persuasive form of evidence on which to base decisions about service developments and investment priorities. The evidence hierarchy is best suited to evaluating evidence relating to the primary prevention of disease and specific health promotion activities, rather than to complex and community based initiatives like community development and regeneration. Gowman and Coote call for a new shared framework of evidence, based around common policy goals and health improvement objectives, and shared beliefs and values about the principles that should inform judgements about different types of evidence. Others policy makers have argued for a similar approach:

There are limitations to both science and practice. Public health science and practice are part of a continuum and it is only by bringing these two strands together that a complete body of knowledge can be developed and public health evidence and capacity be built (Naish 2002).

The impact on the workforce and patient care

Medicine has had a hugely beneficial impact on the lives of millions of patients. Every year new medical advances bring the ability to cure previously untreatable diseases. The history of medicine since the second world war has been called 'one of the most impressive epochs of human achievement' (Le Fanu 1999). Amongst the long list of achievements in the last fifty years can be included the discovery of penicillin, the eradication of small pox, the development of imaging modalities and the first open heart surgery, kidney transplant and test tube baby (Chantler 2002).

However, the dominance of the medical model of health has sometimes had had less positive consequences for the delivery of care. It has been an important factor behind the greater status (and resources) attached to specialist services provided in hospitals rather than to other forms of care. The so called 'Cinderella' services that use teams of practitioners to deliver care within communities, like mental health and social care, are seen as less prestigious or interesting than medicine, offering few merit awards and little private practice (Harrison and Dixon 2000; Salvage 2002).

The medical model of health has also resulted in a lack of resources and priority being given to public health skills. The Royal College of General Practitioners and the Faculty of Public Health Medicine (2001) have suggested that GPs may lack the skills and capacity necessary to deliver their part of the public health function. One study found that whilst GPs often endorse the principle of prevention, many regard it as a low status activity and seek to limit their own personal involvement by delegating it to nurses (Adams *et al* 2001). Whilst often enthusiastic about taking forward public health, nurses and health visitors face their own capacity constraints such as high vacancy rates (Rowe 2002).

The medical model of health has also had specific consequences for the way in which care is provided. One example is the focus of services for mothers and children during the early years of life. The emergence of the community paediatric speciality during the 1970s and 1980s led to a strong emphasis on screening individual children in terms of their growth and development, rather than on providing practical and emotional support for parents, and health visitors have become increasingly focused on this work (Naish 2002). Qualitative research shows health visitors often concentrate on measuring and weighing babies, rather than on providing parents with help and advice (Edwards 2002). This is important, not only because parents feel their needs are not being effectively met but because there is a growing body of evidence that the nature and quality of parents' interactions with their children is a key factor affecting child development (Harker and Kendall 2003). Many health visitors acknowledge this problem, but the evidence suggests they have struggled to move away from ritualised contacts with children and families (Rowe 2002). 'Rules' about professional practice, such as the number of visits to postnatal mothers, and inflexible child health promotion programmes have proved a particular barrier as has the general lack of receptiveness to long term, community based health initiatives from within the NHS (Royal College of Nursing 2002).

The medical model of health has influenced the working practices of all professional groups. For example, it has led to pharmacists focusing on the individual behavioural causes of health inequalities (such as smoking, drinking and poor diet) rather than on understanding the link with wider structural and material factors. It has been suggested that changing this mind set and encouraging pharmacists to think outside the normal confines of the traditional medical model is one of the most important challenges facing the profession. This will require major changes in the way pharmacists are trained, since knowledge about how mortality and morbidity are affected by socio-economic, race, and gender is a minor and sometimes non-existent part of pharmacists' training (Blissell and Jesson 2002).

Whilst the medical profession has gone through substantial changes over recent years, it still exerts a powerful influence on the day to day relationships between doctors and patients and between different professional groups. This report has already referred to the Bristol Royal Infirmary Inquiry which outlined how, at the extreme end of the spectrum, the monopoly of medical power can lead to a failure to disclose malpractice, a failure to heed and act on research findings, and a deep resistance to change. Salvage has argued (2002) that despite the increasing professionalisation of nursing, nurses lack power and influence compared to doctors, and that the basic premise that nurses do what doctors tell them and practise according to what medicine permits, ignores or neglects is still a salient feature of contemporary nursing.

More profound concerns about the consequences of the medical model of health have emerged in recent years. The development of new technologies could accelerate the trend towards the medicalisation of health. Drugs that seek to treat problems which have previously been regarded as non-medical are already on the market. Commentators question whether so-called 'lifestyle' drugs like Viagra for impotence and Xenical for obesity and new neuropharmacological drugs for 'conditions' like shyness, are simply medicalising what are in many cases social, rather than medical problems (New 2000; Wade 2003).

However, there are grounds for being optimistic that doctors may themselves lead the drive for change in future. A recent editorial in the British Medical Journal asked if there is 'too much medicine' in the current system, suggesting that 'increasing medical inputs will at some point become counterproductive and produce more harm than good' (Moynihan and Smith 2002). Other doctors argue the problem goes deeper still, suggesting that the intellectual model of medicine must be changed so that doctors are trained not simply to apply the natural sciences to people's health problems but to become change managers (cited in Smith 2001). Such a shift would have profound consequences not only for undergraduate, graduate and continuing education, but for the health system as a whole.

Integrated and seamless

A key feature of patient-centred care is that it offers seamless, integrated services. This requires effective co-ordination not just within the NHS but between the NHS and other sectors, notably social care. Ensuring that services are seamless and integrated is also crucial to improving safety. As the Institute of Medicine argues (2001):

> It is in inadequate handoffs that safety often fails first. Specifically, in a safe system, information is not lost, inaccessible or forgotten in transitions. Knowledge about patients – such as their allergies, their medications, their diagnostic and treatment plans – is available.

Quantitative and qualitative research of patients' experiences suggests there are currently major difficulties in delivering fully integrated services across all parts of the system. Surveys demonstrate that many patients experience healthcare which is poorly co-ordinated, and that UK patients are more likely to have difficulties than those in other countries. In one study, 37 per cent of patients in the UK said they experienced care that was not well organised, compared to 18 per cent in Switzerland, 20 per cent in Germany and 26 per cent in the US. Eight per cent of UK patients said that doctor/nurse teamwork was not good, compared to 4 per cent in Switzerland, 6 per cent in Germany and 7.5 per cent in the US. In addition, 23 per cent of UK patients said staff gave them conflicting information, compared to 14 per cent in Switzerland, 15 per cent in Germany and 18 per cent in the US (Coulter and Cleary 2001).

Qualitative research supports this analysis. Patients often feel they have to struggle to get all parts of the system to work together effectively and highlight important 'gaps' in their care, such as practitioners not having access to the same information about their condition or treatment plan (Edwards 2001). Greater diversity in the provision of healthcare, through the introduction of Diagnostic and Treatment

Centres and an increased role for the private and non-profit sectors, is likely to make the issue of co-ordinating health services even more challenging in future.

Integrating services across health and social care boundaries is as, if not more, problematic than integrating services within the NHS. Poor co-ordination, particularly of older people's services, has been identified as a major problem by successive reports and inquiries (see for example, Audit Commission 1997; 1999; 2000; 2002). As the population ages, demand for more effective integration of health and social care is likely to increase.

Integrating services within the NHS: the implications of specialisation

A range of factors affect the delivery of integrated services within the NHS. The first is the number of different staff involved in the process of care, which can make effective co-ordination both difficult and time consuming. For example, a study of how x-rays were taken in one hospital calculated that the process involved eleven members of staff, using thirty different processes, and taking 124 minutes to complete (cited in Black and Garside 1994).

This problem is exacerbated by the increasing specialisation of the health workforce. There are now 25 sub-specialities within the general physician specialty, eight sub-specialities within general surgery and five sub-specialities within general pathology. Increasing specialisation is not confined to medicine: the Royal College of Nursing has 80 specialist interest forums. All western healthcare systems are becoming more specialised: there are over 2,000 categories of health professional and over 120 groups of physician/specialists in the US, compared with ten categories of health professionals and twelve categories of medical specialists fifty years ago (Lawrence 2002).

The forces pushing towards greater specialisation include the pace and complexity of technological advance, the evidence linking some measures of quality to greater specialisation (for example in surgical outcomes), concerns about safety, the increase in litigation and the significant growth in direct access services provided by other professions (Wanless 2002). Increasing specialisation is also related to the kudos and status which is afforded to specialist practice, something which has long been the case in medicine but which is increasingly reflected in other areas of the workforce such as nursing and the professions allied to medicine. For example, research suggests that the overlap in the work carried out by occupational therapists and physiotherapists in the community has resulted from a desire to promote and protect professional identity (Smith *et al* 2000).

Greater specialisation can lead to improvements in patient care as knowledge and expertise is refined and concentrated in the hands of specialist practitioners. However, whilst the value of specialist care must not be underestimated, it may also come at a price, including a lack of investment in generalist skills (Royal College of Surgeons 2001) and the poor co-ordination of services (Vaughan 2002). Finding an appropriate balance between generalist and specialist skills has been identified as one of the biggest challenges facing health services in the years ahead (Wanless 2002; Lawrence 2002).

A number of developments have sought to address these issues in recent years. The need to improve co-ordination between different members of the health workforce is an important factor behind the drive towards inter-professional training (Humphris and Macleod Clark 2002). Local initiatives have sought to develop new types of workers whose skills cut across traditional professional divides, in order to help improve the co-ordination of patient care. For example, in some parts of the country the roles of nursing assistants, physiotherapy helpers and occupational therapy helpers have been amalgamated to help improve services for patients with long term rehabilitation needs. In future, multi-skilled generic support workers could help improve the continuity of care provided, tackling professional differences about priorities in care for example by using common care plans.

Some policy makers and practitioners have called for the development of new workers in the professional as well as the support workforce. The Future Healthcare Workforce Group[7] argues that a radical simplification and streamlining of the workforce is vital in order to improve service co-ordination and deliver more patient centred care. Three key groups of staff are proposed to work across traditional professional divides: Specialists (including consultants, GPs, senior registrars and clinical scientists); Health Care Practitioners (combining the skills of nurses, allied health professionals and doctors in training) and Health Care Practitioner Assistants (incorporating the roles of health care assistants, nursing auxiliaries and assistants and helpers to allied health professionals). These practitioners could be used in a range of primary and acute healthcare settings. Developing the new roles would require major changes in the way staff are trained, including direct entry onto education and training programmes (Schofield 1996; Cochrane *et al* 1999; 2002).

The need to clarify roles

Another factor which can inhibit the delivery of seamless services, and which is linked to the proliferation of occupational groups, is the lack of clarity about who does what within the process of care. The working practices of different professional groups are often shrouded in uncertainty and even myth. Such myths are an important mechanism by which some practitioners have both consciously and unconsciously protected their scope of practice and excluded other members of the healthcare team.

The need to improve understanding between different members of the health workforce is a key element in the drive towards inter-professional training. As the report of the Bristol Royal Infirmary Inquiry argues:

> One of the most effective ways to foster an understanding about and respect for various professional roles and the value of multi-professional teams is to expose medical and nursing students, other healthcare professionals and managers to shared education and training (Kennedy *et al* 2001).

Local initiatives have also sought to clarify what happens during the patients' pathway through the system, in order to improve the quality of care being provided. For example, new 'collaborative programmes' have brought together all staff involved in the process of patient care to describe the patient's journey through the system, including nurses, consultants, medical secretaries and technicians. Key 'blockages' or problems are identified, such as gaps in services or areas of duplication. A plan for improving and streamlining the care process is then agreed, which may involve the development of tools like shared assessments and care protocols (Coronary Heart Disease Collaborative 2001).

Collaborative programmes can be hugely challenging to some sections of the workforce. The development of shared assessments and protocols requires staff to accept the systemisation of their practices, and greater transparency and accountability for their actions. This can prompt accusations that a 'cook book' approach to the provision of care is being attempted. Such initiatives can also challenge long held beliefs about the core of the professional's sense of identity. Elements of the medical profession may fear a loss clinical autonomy because of the drive towards working in teams. Parts of the nursing may also fear the 'essence' of their professionalism – something they have fought hard to secure over the years – will be diluted if skills deemed integral to nursing are shared with other members of staff like health care assistants.

However, research suggests these fears can be overcome if clinicians feel ownership over the process of change and can see demonstrable benefits for patients. A recent evaluation of a cancer services collaborative found considerable scepticism to the programme at the initial stage, particularly from consultants, who saw the programme as an administrative initiative rather than an attempt to improve the quality of care. One even claimed it could be 'left to the girls in outpatients'. The threat that mapping the patients' pathway through the system presented to existing power relations was a critical factor in the initial resistance of consultants. However, once practices that consultants themselves called 'absurd' were thrown up by the mapping process, they often became convinced of the need for change.

Thus gaining and maintaining the commitment of all staff, particularly the medical profession, is crucial to success. As one manager interviewed for the cancer collaborative study commented: 'You can have all your managers on board, all your clerks, all your nursing staff and your allied health professionals, but if your consultant staff aren't on board then it ain't going to work' (Gollop 2003).

Integrating health and social care

The difficulties of integrating health and social care services are well known. Poor co-ordination has been repeatedly identified as a major failing in the system, particularly in relation to older people's services. A range of factors contribute to the problem, including the difficulties in aligning boundaries and budgets for service users; the continuing policy of charging for social and 'personal' care but not for health services; the poor development of information management and technology; and persistent prejudices and stereotypes about different professional cultures (Rummery and Glendinning 2000).

Despite the broad nature of the problems associated with effectively co-ordinating health and social care, the predominant policy response has been to focus on structural change. The main thrust of current Government policy, for example, is to encourage the development of Care Trusts: organisations that will commission both health and social care for their local populations. Yet the potential benefits of structural change in improving the integration of health and social care at the front line are far from clear. Only one Care Trust has been the subject of research to date. The results are not encouraging, suggesting the new arrangements have failed to produce significant benefits to users during the first two years (Davies 2002). This echoes evidence from Northern Ireland, which suggests that structural integration is not necessarily an effective means of providing integration at the front line (McCoy 2000).

Changing practices, developing new roles

Wistow (2002) argues that better outcomes for those with health and social care needs will primarily be achieved by changing working practices, rather than by further structural reform. He calls for greater use of integrated care pathways, based on evidence-based protocols, which specify the roles, responsibilities and sequence of interventions by the different professionals involved, along similar lines to the collaborative programmes discussed above.

Other policy makers argue that new practitioners who combine health and social care roles that are currently separate will also need to emerge. Vaughan argues (2002) that elements of nursing, occupational therapy, social work and home support could be drawn together in a new profession focusing on providing services for older people who do not need to be in hospital but would benefit from other types of care such as rehabilitation or recuperation (sometimes referred to as intermediate care). The needs of this group are not currently being adequately met: recent estimates suggest 29 per cent of people occupying acute hospital beds have needs that are not commensurate with that level of care, including 34 per cent who require home or bed-based recuperation and 6 per cent who require more complex rehabilitation (Vaughan and Withers 2002).

The Future Healthcare Workforce Group argues that new Health Care Practitioners should largely replace the wide range of staff groups who currently work with older people, including district nurses, physiotherapists, occupational therapists, speech and language therapists and care managers. The main elements of the Health Care Practitioners' role would be taking a comprehensive health and social care history, physical examination and diagnosis, developing and implementing care plans, co-ordinating services across health and social care settings, evaluating users responses to care, health promotion and education and research and audit. New Health Practitioner Assistants (incorporating the role of healthcare assistants, helpers to physiotherapists and elements of the care assistant role) would be the main point of contact for patients. They would play an important role in implementing the care plan, both in inpatient units and in the patient's home, carrying out investigative procedures (within clear parameters) such as taking blood samples and ECGs, and liasing with other agency's to co-ordinate services like shopping or providing meals (Cochrane 2002). However, developing these new practitioners would require major changes in the way the future health and social care workforce is trained and tackling disparities in the pay levels of the health and social care sectors.

A holistic model of care

Wider changes may be necessary if health and social care services are to be effectively integrated in future. The organisation and delivery of care will need to be based on a more holistic model of health (an issue this report has already explored). Wistow (2002) uses the example of a safe discharge from hospital to illustrate this point. From a purely medical perspective, a safe discharge would be one that is clinically safe, in other words the person would be physically capable of moving back home. However, a non-clinical perspective would lead to the consideration of other issues such as the person's social needs, for example whether they have a safe home and community to return to. Wistow argues that providing genuinely holistic care means addressing people's emotional and psychological needs, as well as their physical and medical ones. Research suggests that over a third of people living in the community five years after having survived a stroke suffer from depression and between a third and a half of their carers also suffer from depression. Stroke care based on restricted definitions of need is therefore likely to lead to poor quality outcomes for individuals and their carers (Wilkinson *et al* 1997; Han and Haley 1998; Wistow 2002).

Developing a more holistic understanding of users needs has major implications for the way needs are assessed, the way services are organised, developed and performance managed, and how the workforce is planned, trained and remunerated. As Vaughan explains (in relation to the provision of intermediate care):

> Traditionally patient care is packaged on the basis of clinical diagnosis. Access is provided through diagnostically grouped clinical teams and funding in acute care follows completed consultant episodes. By contrast, intermediate care services are founded on a model of health care that shifts from definition of treatment by medical diagnosis to a needs related service... The shift that is advocated is not just an organisational change but a major alteration in culture that moves away from the traditional paradigm from which health care has been developed to a broader based model, built on a mix of health and social well being (Vaughan 2002).

Informing and empowering

Poor communication and a lack of information

One of the biggest challenges facing the NHS is the need to provide more and better quality information for patients. Quantitative research suggests failures in communication are the most frequent source of patient dissatisfaction (Coulter and Cleary 2001; Grol *et al* 2000). Patients suffer from poor communication and a lack of information in all health care systems, but this may be a particular problem in the UK. In one survey, 28 per cent of UK patients said their doctor did not answer their questions clearly, compared to 11 per cent in Switzerland, 17 per cent in Germany and 21 per cent in the US; 34 per cent of UK patients said their test results were not clearly explained to them, compared to 26 per cent in Switzerland, 32 per cent in Germany and 26 per cent in the US; and 38.5 per cent of patients said their family was not given the information that was necessary to help with their recovery, compared to 17 per cent in Switzerland, 28 per cent in Germany and 26 per cent in the US. The survey also found that more than half of UK patients said they received insufficient information in Accident and Emergency, compared to 28 per cent in Switzerland, 32 per cent in Germany and 40 per cent in the US (Coulter and Cleary 2002).

Qualitative research supports these findings (Edwards 2001). Patients generally feel very ill informed in today's NHS. This lack of information is apparent at every level of the patient's experience: from not knowing what is going to happen to them when they go into hospital and how long their treatment will take, to a lack of information about the purpose and potential side effects of medicines. Finding out what is often very basic information is one of the main 'battles' patients struggle to cope with in their contact with the health service (Kendall 2001). Poor communication and the lack of information given to patients are thought to be one of the main factors underlying the rising number of complaints in the NHS: 28,000 people make written complaints about aspects of their treatment in hospitals each year (Fishwick and Letts 2002). These figures may be the tip of the iceberg: around two-thirds of people who say they would have liked to comment or complain about their health care do not pursue their concerns (National Consumer Council 1998).

Whilst today's patients don't get enough information, tomorrow's may suffer the opposite problem (Pyper 2002). One of the main reasons for this is the explosion of information available via the internet. There are currently around 10,000 health information websites and the number of new health websites in the EU is increasing by 300 per month (Wanless 2001). However, the quality of information available on many of these sites is questionable (Risk and Dzenowagis 2001) – something which patients themselves recognise and express concern about (Edwards 2001). The need to tackle social inequalities in access to information on the internet (the so-called 'digital divide') and to provide health information that is relevant at the local level is a key challenge in the years ahead (Pyper 2002).

Lack of patient involvement

Empowering patients is not simply about providing them with good quality, relevant information. It is also about ensuring that those patients who want to can use this information to participate in decisions about their own treatment and care. Research shows that sharing decisions with patients can leader to better outcomes and a reduction in patient anxiety and depression, as well as improved satisfaction rates (Coulter *et al* 1999).

However, surveys suggest that the majority of patients do not feel they are given enough of a say in their treatment at present, with UK patients feeling far less involved than those in other countries. In one survey, 60 per cent of UK patients said they didn't have enough of a say in their treatment, compared with 36 per cent of patients in Switzerland, 46 per cent in Germany and 37 per cent in the US (Coulter and Cleary 2002). Whilst the desire for greater involvement in decisions is high across all groups, it can be influenced by cultural factors (Coulter 2002); age – with younger patients being more likely to want greater involvement than older patients (Edwards 2001); and the stage of the patients' condition – for example those with serious conditions like cancer may express a greater desire for guidance at the early stages of diagnosis (Cassileth *et al* 1980).

Involving patients can mean more than sharing decisions about treatment options. Patients have an important role to play in 'self-caring' for common and minor conditions. One study of over 500 people found that a substantial proportion already take on considerable responsibilities for self care: around half of the illness episodes recorded by the patients during a four week period resulted in self-care activities alone, 17 per cent resulted in self care and professional care and five per cent in professional care alone (Rogers *et al* 1999). Yet despite the evidence that many patients already conduct some forms of self-care, patients often fail to see a role for themselves beyond 'doing what they are told' (Edwards 2001). Patients are often unaware how long common ailments or conditions might be expected to last. The cost of over the counter medicines, particularly for disadvantaged patients, is another barrier to more widespread practice of self-care (Kendall 2001).

There is also growing interest in how patients with long-term illnesses can be supported to take on responsibility for managing certain aspects of their condition. Research has demonstrated that self-management programmes can make a major contribution to improving health outcomes. Patients who have participated in Chronic Disease Self-Management Courses have been shown to experience an increase in self-efficiency (perception of disease control), reduced distress and fatigue, improved symptom control and better mental health (Fishwick and Letts,2002). Evidence demonstrates that educational interventions which enhance people's self-efficacy can also help reduce demand for medical interventions, leading to cost savings (Vickery and Lynch 1995). Asthma patients who participate in self-management programmes have been shown to pay fewer visits to their GP and to Accident and Emergency departments and spend less overall time in hospital (Cooper 2001a).

Programmes like these will become increasingly important as the population ages and more people live with chronic conditions. Professional organisations have acknowledged the critical role that patients can play in the process of care. The new Code of Professional Conduct for nurses specifically recognises that patients are partners in their own care and that patients, their carers and wider family should be seen as key members of the health care 'team' (Nursing and Midwifery Council 2002). The Government has also recognised the need to improve support for people with long-term illnesses and established an Expert Patient programme to encourage the development of self-management programme throughout all areas of the NHS by 2007. However, only £3 million has been invested in the initiative so far – a drop in the ocean compared to the scale of the task at hand.[8]

Implications for services, practitioners and patients

A major barrier to effective communication between professionals and patients is the lack of time available during consultations (Williams et al 1998). Research suggests that 20 minute consultations are needed to effectively involve patients in decisions about treatment, give them a sense of control and enable them to take on responsibility for some aspects of their care (Kaplan et al 1995). Yet time is a rare commodity in the NHS, particularly in primary care – something which is keenly felt by patients and professionals alike (Kendall 2001).

Changes in practitioners' relationships with patients will be critical if patients are to be effectively empowered. A more informed and educated population and the decline in social deference means patients are increasingly inclined to question health professionals. Technological advances have re-enforced this trend. As Muir Gray (1999) argues: 'the world wide web, the dominant medium of the post modern world, has blown away the doors and walls of the locked library as effectively as semtex.' These developments can challenge what many practitioners believe to be at the heart of their professionalism: being the sole possessor of a unique body of knowledge and expertise.

Many doctors have already recognised that they are no longer the only creators or custodians of the knowledge base and that their role will increasingly be to help guide, interpret and explain information to patients. This will require doctors to be more honest with patients, and to share risks and admit mistakes (Irvine 2002). However, greater honesty and transparency will be crucial to building trust with clinicians (and the health system as a whole):

> One important route to restoring trust is through a commitment to transparency by all healthcare systems. Organisations and clinicians that act as thought they have nothing to hide become more trustworthy. The healthcare system should seek to earn renewed trust not by hiding its defects but by revealing them along with making a relentless commitment to improve (Institute of Medicine 2001).

The process of informing patients, involving them in decisions and sharing risks is highly complex. Some patients may wish to avoid risk, others may choose a risky intervention despite a relatively low likelihood of benefit. Patients' preferences are likely to change over time and to depend on the clinical problems in question. The enterprise of shared decision making is a dynamic one, changing as patients and circumstances change (Institute of Medicine 2001).

New skills

Practitioners will need a wide range of skills to fulfil this role in future, including the ability to explore the patient's ideas about the problem, finding out the patient's preferred role in the process, describing treatment options, providing tailor-made information to the patient, ensuring the patient understands the information, and then helping the patient to interpret the evidence and risk (Elwyn *et al* 2000).

The professions and government have recognised the need to improve the way practitioners communicate with their patients. The GMC has made communication skills the highest priority for the five year validation reports for existing doctors. Communication skills are also becoming a core part of undergraduate training for every new health professional (Department of Health 2000a). However, concerns about the effectiveness of this training have already been raised. The evidence suggests that whilst professional educators understand the importance of imparting a patient-centred approach to their students, when asked what this would involve in practice, the focus tends to be on topics such as how to break bad news or explain technical procedures to patients rather than on establishing a genuine dialogue between patients and professionals or increasing patient autonomy (Gillespie *et al* 2002). Thus for too many health professionals, communicating with patients remains focused on telling and instructing: 'rather than helping to create circumstances in which individuals attain emotional and intellectual insight into the fact that the quality of the rest of their lives will largely be determined by their own efforts' (Taylor 2001). For example, research into the way information and education for asthma patients is provided shows that professionals tend to concentrate on what they believe patients need to know, such as the basic mechanisms of disease and the correct choice of drugs, rather than the skills that patients need to help them become effective managers of their condition (Clark and Gong 2000).

This problem is related to the medical model of health within which many practitioners work and to which this report has already referred. Professionals tend to see patients needs for information from a purely medical perspective whereas patients want information which takes their whole needs into account (Gillespie *et al* 2002). However, doctors' failure to communicate effectively with patients is also related to patients' reluctance to share the risks and problems associated with medicine and healthcare, as well as its potential benefits. In future, patients' roles will need to evolve as much as doctors'. Patients need to understand the limits to modern medicine, as well as its capacity to bring about change. Patients' current lack of understanding is in part a consequence of professionals refusing to share information and discuss risks in the past. It is only by establishing a new relationship between doctors and patients that this impasse can be overcome. This new relationship will be vital in delivering other key characteristics of patient-centred care, particularly improving patient safety and shifting away from a culture of blame (Institute of Medicine 2001). The need for a 'sea change' in the attitudes of both health professionals and patients is now clear. Achieving this change will require radical changes in the way health professionals are trained. It will also mean finding new ways of shaping patient-professional relationships. The British Medical Journal has recently called for that a new 'contract' between patients and doctors, where doctors share much greater information with patients but that patients begin to understand the risks (Smith 2001). This might take the shape of a general understanding, but it could also take a more concrete form, involving a specific set of rights and responsibilities negotiated between patients, their doctors and other members of the health team. Such a contract might be particularly appropriate for patients with long-term conditions, since their role in the process of care is integral to improving health outcomes.

Timely and convenient

Quicker, more flexible access

The speed with which people can access health services is patients' top priority and one of the main sources of current dissatisfaction with the NHS (Kendall 2001). The National Survey of NHS Patients indicates that the highest levels of patient discontent are about accessing GP services and waiting times for hospital appointments and treatment (Department of Health 1998). Qualitative research supports this analysis, suggesting that by far the most frustrating experience of the NHS is that of waiting: waiting for a doctor's appointment, waiting for an appointment with a specialist or consultant, waiting in the doctor's surgery or hospital once patients have an appointment, and then waiting to be discharged (Kendall 2001).

People also want more flexible access to healthcare. Patients want access to the GP's surgery outside traditional working hours both in the evenings and during the weekends (Cabinet Office 2000). One of the main reasons why people want after-hours access to public services is that they do not like managing their personal business at work. Wider changes in society, such as the increasing number of mothers with young children entering the workplace, mean it is often difficult for people to attend appointments during office hours.

Providing quicker, more convenient services is clearly important in terms of improving individual patients' satisfaction with their experience. For patients, waiting means being out of control, getting anxious, wasting time and generally feeling unimportant (Edwards 2001). Improving access to health services may also be critical to retaining public support for the NHS as a whole. There is evidence that patients are beginning to compare the service they receive from the NHS with services available on the high street (Edwards and Clark 2001). Both the private sector and other comparable health care systems are seen as being more responsive to their patients than the NHS (McKinsey and Company 2001).

A publicly funded service must seek to respond to the changing aspirations of the society it seeks to serve, if it is to retain sufficient support over the long term. However, the NHS is not just another consumer organisation: it is a public service with a different purpose and set of objectives, and rightly so. Encouraging patients to view the NHS from a purely consumerist perspective will lead to inevitable dissatisfaction since there will always be difficult trade-offs between the needs of individual patients and those of the wider community (Kendall 2001).

Ensuring patients have timely access to health care is not just about increasing patient satisfaction – it is also crucial to improving health outcomes. Too many patients are currently reaching a dangerously advanced stage of disease by the time they are treated (Wanless 2001). More than a third of people who have been referred to a hospital doctor by their GP say their condition worsens whilst waiting for the appointment. Over half say they are in pain during this time and that their condition limits their work or daily activities (Department of Health 1998). If inappropriately long waits for treatment cause complications with the patient's condition, it not only harms the individual's health but also the overall cost-effectiveness of the system. Difficulties in accessing GPs can result in-patients going to Accident and Emergency departments to receive care. Treating patients in hospital who do not need acute care, particularly in accident and emergency, can delay the treatment of those in greater need and is also more expensive that providing care at the primary care level.

Increasing capacity, changing roles

The Government has set a series of ambitious targets to cut waiting times. By 2004 patients should be able to have a GP's appointment within 24 hours and by the end of 2005, the maximum wait for an outpatient appointment should be three months and for an inpatient appointment, six months (Department of Health 2000a).

Professionals and managers have expressed concern about whether these targets are either appropriate, because of the perverse incentives they can create, or achievable within the given timescale. The main problem is the severe capacity constraints which continue to bedevil the NHS, despite the substantial increases in spending which are now going into the system. Primary amongst these constraints are the staff shortages being faced in the NHS. Shortages are now being experienced across all occupational groups, from consultants to GPs, and from nurses to the allied health professions (see for example Department of Health 2002a). These shortages and have been emphasised by the introduction of the European Working Time Directive to reduce junior doctors' hours.

A major focus of government policy is therefore to increase the number of staff. The NHS Plan set targets to provide an extra 7,500 consultants, 2,000 GPs, 20,000 nurses and 6,500 therapists (Department of Health 2000a). Strategies for achieving these targets include increasing the number of staff from overseas, running a series of recruitment campaigns, providing incentives to encourage staff to enter the system ('golden hellos') and to encourage existing staff to stay ('golden goodbyes'). A series of initiatives to help improve retention rates for example through improving childcare facilities and encouraging family friendly working are also being implemented.

The Government has made considerable progress towards meeting its targets for increasing staff numbers, particularly nurses. However, professional organisations and trades unions have criticised the Government's targets for being based on headcount figures, rather than whole time equivalents, arguing that these will be insufficient to deliver the commitments set out in the NHS Plan. A number of trends are likely to put more pressure on staff numbers in future. The nursing workforce is ageing: the number of nurses forecast to retire will double from 5,500 a year to more than 10,000 a year by 2005. Significant numbers of

Asian GPs who were recruited to plug gaps in the 1970s are now approaching retirement. While the number of places in medical school are increasing, the number of applicants is falling (Appleby and Coote 2002), something which may be exacerbated by recent changes to the financing of higher education. These pressures suggest that increasing the capacity of the NHS workforce will depend as much on changing the roles and responsibilities of health workers as on increasing their overall number. Policies to change what practitioners do and where and how they work are going with the grain of change. Capacity constraints, combined with the changing aspirations of staff, have led to a whole range of practitioners extending their scope of practice over recent years.

Improving access to secondary care

Whilst there have been changes in the working practices of staff across the health sector, there has tended to be a greater focus on developing roles in secondary care, rather than in primary care or across the health and social care sectors. This is for a number of reasons, including the generally greater priority given to healthcare policy in the acute sector, the higher costs associated with staff in secondary care, and the fact that GPs have traditionally exerted considerable influence over developments in staff roles in primary care.

Changing roles for doctors

One of the most important areas where doctors working practices have change in recent years is in the expanded use of day surgery. New techniques of minimal access surgery allow surgeons to perform microscopic and macroscopic operations in places which formerly could only be reached via large incisions, reducing the physical and psychological trauma associated with open wound surgery (Darzi 1999).

Since the early 1990s the use of day surgery for many procedures has grown. However, a report from the Audit Commission (2001) suggests that if all trusts achieved the levels of the best performers, 120,000 existing inpatients in England and Wales could be treated as day cases. The report cites inguinal hernia repair as a typical example where Trusts range between treating none and 80 per cent of their patients as day cases. The increasing use of day surgery units for inpatient work (particularly during times of 'winter pressure') is a crucial factor underlying these variations. The Government has recognised this problem and is introducing a range of new Diagnosis and Treatment Centres (DTCs) to provide low risk, high volume elective surgery and diagnostic procedures. The aim is for DTCs to be staffed by dedicated surgeons, nurses and support staff whose work is unaffected by seasonal and emergency demands.

The evidence suggests that professional attitudes and working practices play a critical role in determining the amount of day surgery that takes place. Clinicians may be reluctant to accept that some procedures are suitable for day surgery, despite the evidence from best practice. There are also wide variations in staff productivity rates between units. Many factors can affect productivity, including the grade mix of staff and the degree of clerical support (Audit Commission 2001).

There has been surprisingly little research on the productivity rates of surgeons to date. The first major study conducted for the Department of Health demonstrated substantial variations between individual surgeons. A number of reasons for these differences have been put forward, including variations in capacity constraints (inadequate levels of nursing or bed shortages), differences between the amount of time surgeons spend working for the British Medical Association and the Royal College (for example examining or doing scientific work), and different levels of private practice (Bloor and Maynard 2002). More effective use of information like this will be critical if access to secondary care is to be improved in future.

Expanding nurses roles

Nurses are taking on a range of extra roles and responsibilities in secondary care as nurse practitioners, nurse consultants and clinical nurse specialists. These developments have played a vital role in reducing doctors' workloads: evidence from the Royal College of Physicians suggests that extending nurses' roles has also been the single most important measure allowing progress towards meeting the EU Directive on junior doctors' working hours (Royal College of Physicians 2001).

Evaluations show that new roles for nurses have helped provide more timely and convenient care. A study of a clinical nurse specialist performing biopsies for a cancer team demonstrated a reduction in waiting times between referral and biopsy from eight weeks to the same day (Kenny 2002). Extending nurses' roles can bring additional benefits. For example, randomised controlled trials which have directly compared nurse practitioners with doctors have shown that nurse practitioners in secondary care score better on communication than doctors (Sakr *et al* 1999; Cooper 2001b); and that clinical nurse specialist interventions for patients experiencing chronic heart failure lead to improved outcomes for patients (Blue *et al* 2001).

It is clear that expanded roles for nurses can help reduce doctors' workloads, cut waiting times and deliver high quality care. Building on these benefits in future means ensuring nurses do not become overburdened themselves. Nursing shortages have already increased attention on the contribution made by non-professionally qualified staff. Studies indicate that health care assistants often carry out complex tasks in the process of patient care (Ramprogus and O'Brien 2002) and act as the patient's advocate within the health care system (Thornely 1998) – roles that have been traditionally conducted by nurses. However, the contribution that non-professionally qualified staff make to the delivery of patient care has not been well recognised and the training needs of this section of the workforce have been a particularly neglected issue to date (Rogers 2002).

Changing roles in primary care

Nurses

One of the most prominent examples of the way in which roles are changing is the increasing use of nurses as the 'first port of call' in primary care. Nurses are now assessing and giving advice to patients with minor conditions through the NHS Direct telephone line and NHS Walk in Centres. Many of the 20,000 nurse prescribers and nurse practitioners who provide independent diagnosis and treatment for patients are based in primary care. Nurses are also leading a number of Primary Medical Service (PMS) pilot schemes. PMS, introduced under the 1997 NHS (Primary Care) Act, enables general medical and dental services to be delivered by directly employed doctors and nurses according to locally negotiated agreements, rather than through the traditional arrangement where independent GPs deliver General Medical

Services under a nationally negotiated GP contract. A range of different arrangements emerged from the first wave of nurse-led PMS pilots. In some schemes, nurses became independent contractors, employing other staff including the GP and those working on reception. In one area, the nurse and all the other members of the practice were salaried, with the nurse acting as the team leader, accountable for the development of services within the practice. In another area, the nurse and GP acted as equal partners in the delivery of patient care (Jones 2000).

Research suggests that the expansion of nurses' roles in primary care has helped deliver higher levels of patient satisfaction and a quality of care that is at least as good as, if not better than, that provided by doctors (Horrocks *et al* 2002). New roles have been linked to the provision of more timely and convenient care: for example a study of a minor surgery nurse practitioner in primary care indicated a reduction in typical waiting times for evening clinics (Martin 2002). Randomised controlled trails of nurse practitioners in primary care have shown that nurses offer more advice on self-care and the self management of conditions than GPs (Shum *et al* 2000; Kinnersley *et al* 2000). Research suggests that patients both accept and welcome the expanded role for nurses in nurse-led PMS schemes. The amount of time the nurse spends with patients, and the social support and continuity of care the nurse provides are key factors in the high levels of satisfaction and confidence expressed by patients (Chapple *et al* 2000).

Doctors' attitudes towards expanding nurse roles have had an important influence on their implementation. Evaluations of nurse led PMS schemes found that whilst some medics 'championed' the pilots, others were less than supportive: several nurse practitioners reported that consultants were sceptical about their referrals, sometimes refusing to accept them (Lewis 2001). Qualitative research with GPs about the role of nurse practitioners reveals GPs can perceive the role as threatening their status, including their job and financial security. GPs also question nurses' capabilities and the quality of their training (Wilson *et al* 2002).

Professional attitudes are not the only barrier to extending nurses roles. Nurse practitioners have reported a lack of training and support for their new roles, including from their professional bodies (Lewis 2001). The current legislative framework also places limitations on nurses' ability to independently manage nurse-led PMS schemes.

Specific barriers include the fact that patients must register with a doctor, that GPs must sign virtually all prescriptions, that there are restrictions on nurses' powers to provide certification for example in the case of death or mental health sectioning or in singing notes confirming patients absence from work due to sickness (Jones 1999). This degree of restriction contrasts with the US, where nurse practitioners practise without any requirement for physician supervision or collaboration in 50 per cent of states (Mudinger *et al* 2000).

The new GPs contract may help to address some of these problems, for example by allowing patients to register with their local practice, rather than with an individual doctor. However, ensuring there is wider acceptance of nurses' position as clinical leaders, improving training and support, and addressing legal barriers will be crucial if nurses roles in primary care are to be further developed in future (Lewis 2001).

Pharmacists

The scope for pharmacists to help reduce GPs' workloads has long been recognised (Nuffield Foundation 1986). It has been suggested that nearly 2.75 million hours of doctors' time could be saved if pharmacists were responsible for dispensing by instalments prescriptions for patients with long-term conditions (Department of Health 2002b). Evidence indicates that pharmacists can also help reduce minor injuries as a proportion of GPs' workloads by taking on responsibility for their management (Hassell *et al* 2001).

A number of recent initiatives have sought to expand pharmacists' roles. An extension of prescribing rights means that pharmacists will be able to prescribe a wider range of medicines on the basis of guidelines developed in conjunction with doctors. This extension could save around 2.5 million GP appointments for the treatment of minor injuries and ailments. Pharmacists are also initiating early detection programmes, running awareness campaigns and advising on rational, safe prescribing policies (Murdock 2002).

In future, pharmacists' roles could expand further still. Instead of having to collect repeat prescriptions from the GP and take them to the pharmacy, patients with long term conditions (of whom there will be an increasing proportion) could be contacted directly by the pharmacist when they need their medicine or even visited at home. Pharmacists could also monitor patients' health status, check for adverse drug reactions and screen for previously undiagnosed conditions using new genetic tests. These developments could help not only reduce GPs' workloads and ensure pharmacists' make better use of their skills, but lead to improvements in the overall cost-effectiveness of the system and shift the focus of services more towards prevention (Murdock 2002). Yet the ability of pharmacists to take on new roles is far from assured. Pharmacists have been anxious about increasing their responsibilities in the past (Blenkinsopp and Bradley 1996). This is partly because they are concerned about making mistakes, but also because they are facing an increasing workload in future. The 'fallow year' created when the pharmacy undergraduate course was extended from three to four years, alongside the predicted increase in the volume of prescriptions over the next five years by 33 per cent (driven in part by the introduction of National Service Frameworks) has stretched the pharmacy workforce. Delays in the implementation of Electronic Patient Records, and disputes about how these should best be developed, are another factor preventing pharmacists from fully developing their roles, as is the way pharmacists are paid. The existing system mainly provides for the physical dispensing of prescriptions rather than broader roles such as screening for conditions or advising patients about how to self-care (Murdock 2002).

Shifting care out of hospitals

Another element of the Government's strategy to reduce waiting times and provide more convenient access to care is to move services out of secondary care and into the local community, where this is appropriate and effective.

The Government plans to create 1,000 General Practitioners with a Specialist Interest (GPSI) by 2004 (Department of Health 2000a). GPSI aim to improve access to care at a location close to the patient whilst also giving specialist support to the wider primary health community (Williams et al 2002). For example, GPSI in Bradford now carry out minor surgery, almost all elective endoscopy, gastroscopy and cystoscopy, a wide range of chronic disease management and extensive triage work. The introduction of this intermediate level of care by GPSI has led to a fall in endoscopy waits from six to seven months to two to three weeks and in neurology from 49 weeks to five. Whether it is primary or secondary care clinicians who lead the development of GPSI, services has so far varied according to the condition and problem at hand. In Bradford, the development of GPSI has been led by secondary care with the focus being on freeing hospital clinicians up to deal with more complex problems. In Plymouth, a GPSI with specific responsibility for coronary heart disease has been established and is now responsible for leading the pulmonary rehabilitation team across primary and secondary care.

GPSI are at an early stage in their development. However, initial evidence indicates they are helping to improve access to services. For example, evaluations show 30 to 40 per cent of patients with ear, nose and throat (ENT) problems who are usually referred to secondary care can be seen by a GPSI. Non-attendance rates are typically 1 to 2 per cent in GPSI clinics, compared to 11 per cent in ENT outpatient clinics, and patients who see a GPSI need fewer follow up appointments than patients seen in secondary care. What is less clear is whether the development of GPSI will reduce or increase demand in the long run, by revealing previously unmet need. Evaluations show that whilst recently established specialist GPs in ENT have not led to increases in demand, one GPSI who has been in place for more than three years is generating 33 per cent more referrals per 10,000 population than in areas without a specialist GP (Sanderson *et al* 2003).

Engaging secondary care clinicians is a critical factor determining the success of GPSI. Whilst some consultants welcome the development of GPSI, others are less supportive, with reports that some consultants 'feel strongly that the Specialist GPs undermine the ENT profession and promote second class care' (Sanderson *et al* 2003). Important issues include the need to develop referral protocols which are agreed by the GPSI and the consultant, and to establish clear guidelines for accessing beds. Some GPSI are currently trained and accredited by local hospital consultants. However, the Royal College of General Practice is working to establish external standards for GPSI and develop appropriate post-graduate education. A potentially contentious issue is how much GPSI should be paid in relation to hospital consultants. If GPSI are paid too little, the danger is they could be seen as inferior to hospital doctors and lack credibility and status as a result. However, if GPSI are paid too much, it could cause resentment amongst consultants and raise important questions about the cost effectiveness of the system.

Despite these initiatives, the challenges associated with shifting services out of hospitals and into primary care remain considerable. Primary care has traditionally been weaker than secondary care, although successive governments have sought to give more power and resources to those working at the primary care level. The current Government is devolving 75 per cent of the NHS budget to Primary Care Trusts in order to drive change within the system (although the degree to which PCTs will be free to spend this money according to their own priorities rather than national targets is open to question). As this report has already suggested, the relative power of different structures within the NHS is related to longstanding differences in professional status and hierarchy. Unless these issues are tackled, shifting power to primary care may remain a pipedream.

Home care

Future technological developments may help open up the possibility of more care being delivered in local communities, and even in patients' homes. New testing kits will enable chronic diseases to be monitored at home, such as measuring blood glucose for diabetes, peak flow rate for asthma and blood pressure and cholesterol for heart disease. Developments in information technologies like telemedicine will further increase opportunities for home based care, enabling patients to receive treatment and advice from specialists in their own home (Wyatt 2002).

Some commentators suggest that the expectations of both professionals and patients will move from a presumption that inpatient treatment is the norm to the view that patients should be treated in their own home wherever possible. At its boldest, this may result in a 'home first' standard where all health services are delivered in the patient's normal place of residence unless certain factors apply. Such services would require a substantial home support workforce, which would integrate both health and social care, backed up by rapid response units (McClimont 2002).

Whilst ambitious, this approach is by no means beyond the realm of possibility. 'Hospital at home' schemes to treat patients with chronic obstructive pulmonary disease – which accounts for one tenth of all acute medical admissions in Great Britain and is projected to rise in future (Kendrick 1994) – are already running in 16 per cent of all respiratory departments in Great Britain (Johnson *et al* 2001). In these schemes, patients who would usually be managed in hospital have at least part of their care undertaken by nurses who visit them at home. Randomised controlled trials show that days in hospital can be reduced without an adverse effect on clinical outcomes and are accompanied by high levels of patient satisfaction and reductions in cost (Cotton *et al* 2000; Swarska *et al* 2000; Davies *et al* 1999). Delivering this type of integrated home care and medical support implies much closer integration of the health and social care workforce. It also requires the overall position of non-professionally qualified staff within the system, and the lack of policy focus and investment in training they have been afforded to date, to be urgently addressed.

Redefining access?

It future, we may need to re-define what we mean by access to health services. The Institute of Medicine has called for a new 'rule' of continuous access to information, care and support, 24 hours a day, 365 days a year. This would not necessarily imply more visits to see health practitioners, but better use of different means of communicating with patients, for example by e-mail and telephone, and better provision of health information, ranging from the patients' medical record to information about conditions and treatments (Institute of Medicine 2001).

Redefining access in this way has important implications for health practitioners and the NHS as a whole. It has been suggested that telecaring (delivering responsive, high quality services to remote patients using the most appropriate and accepted communications media, colleagues and information sources) could become a key element of the work of both generalist and specialist professionals. This would mean major changes to pre-registration and continuing education (Wyatt 2002).

The technology now exists to provide many alternatives to face-to-face visits. However, its use has not been adapted as a routine part of health practitioners' work. This is partly a result of the poor design of, and under-investment in, the NHS information infrastructure. The health care sector spends less per employee on IT than any other sector of the UK economy. The NHS also spends less on IT than other countries: spending on IT constitutes around 1.5 percent of total heath spending in the UK, compared with around 6 per cent in the US (Wanless 2001). However, professional attitudes may be as important a barrier to the effective use of IT in the NHS as levels of spending. Practitioners, especially doctors, question whether the use of new information technologies is clinically and cost-effective, and fear it could lead to substantial increases in their workload. There is some evidence that use of information technology like emails and telephone consultations could help improve health outcomes and patient satisfaction rates. However, there is an overall lack of evidence in this area which will need to be addressed if new ways of accessing and providing services are to be effectively developed in future (Wyatt 2002).

4. The way forward

This report has argued that the cultures, attitudes and working practices of NHS staff – their relationships with one another, with practitioners in sectors outside the NHS (such as social care) and with patients – play a critical role in determining the quality of healthcare being provided. However, successive governments have focused more on changing the structures of the NHS than on reforming these workforce practices or relationships. Any government that is serious about improving the quality of care must make these issues a priority in future.

The analysis outlined in the previous chapter suggests that where workforce reforms have taken place, they have tended to focus on short term goals such as improving patient safety and making access to services more timely and convenient. Far less attention has been paid to how workforce reforms might contribute to equally important characteristics of patient-centred care, such as promoting and restoring health and informing and empowering patients. More fundamental changes to the workforce will therefore be necessary in order to deliver genuinely patient-centred care in future.

There are four key challenges which need to be addressed:

- *Improving relations between clinicians and managers.* The evidence shows that the key to successfully reforming working practices and services is engaging clinicians, particularly doctors, and demonstrating direct improvements to patient care. A substantial proportion of clinicians feel they lack power and control in today's NHS. Many feel that the Government's targets are at best irrelevant and at worst, a distortion of real clinical priorities. Measures must be taken to more effectively involve clinicians in managing the process of reform at all levels of the NHS. The Government should not seek to impose a 'one size fits all' approach to reforming the future health workforce. Instead, it should focus on making good its promise to cede power and control to the local level and concentrate on removing potential barriers to change so that different models can emerge on the ground.

- *Ensuring closer working between practitioners and sectors.* Many of the key features of patient-centred care rely on closer working between different members of the health team. This suggests that a shift in culture towards a new professionalism, based on shared practice, knowledge and values is required, in contrast to the traditional model of professionalism which emphasises the differences between professions through separate systems of regulation, pay and education.

- *Transforming practitioner-patient relations.* Practitioners must not only effectively inform and involve patients in treatment decisions, but also enable them to take on appropriate responsibilities for their own wellbeing and care. This will require major changes in the roles of practitioners and patients alike.

- *Addressing the dominance of the medical model of health.* Patient centred-care must seek to prevent ill health, and promote and restore good health. It must take a whole person perspective, addressing people's social and emotional needs as well as their physical and medical ones. The dominance of the medical model of health, as well as the short-termism of politics and policy making, have been key factors in the failure of services to achieve these goals to date. Future trends, such as the ageing population and the increasing proportion of people living with chronic conditions, means addressing these issues will be even more important in the years ahead.

In addition, more attention must be paid to evaluating whether workforce reforms deliver genuinely patient-centred care. Too often changes in the workforce are evaluated to assess whether they are cost-effective or if they are acceptable to existing professional groups: patients' views are rarely taken into account (Kendall 2001). If the overall objective of workforce reform is to deliver high quality, patient-centred care, as this report has argued, then patients' views must be integral to the evaluation process.

A new professionalism

Calls for a 'new professionalism' in healthcare have gathered momentum over recent years both in this country and others, notably the US. The concept is still at a formative stage: there are many views about what the 'new professionalism' is, how it differs from previous forms, and how it should be translated in practice.

Davies (1996) has identified several distinctive strands of the new professionalism. The first is that it is based on the notion of interdependency and shared accountability between professions rather than on individual autonomy and accountability. The second, building on the theme of interdependence, is that the new professionalism is inclusive, recognising the contribution of all members of the team to the process of healthcare:

> Recognising the contribution of others to health and healing means much more than doctors acknowledging that nurses or physiotherapists do a good job. It requires a fundamental redefinition of the knowledge base of health care. Valuing the contribution of all means expanding an understanding of health care's boundaries far beyond the traditional confines of scientific medicine (Salvage 2002).

An important element of the inclusiveness which marks out the new professionalism is that certain approaches, skills and values are, or should be, shared by all those entering the health (and potentially social care) professions and that these shared approaches define a health professional.

The third strand of the new professionalism concerns the relationship between practitioners and patients. The practitioners' role and identity should be based on a desire to teach, facilitate and share control with patients rather than to maintain their exclusive mastery of a specific body of knowledge. The final characteristic of the new professionalism is the

---

Table 4.1 Old and new concepts of professionalism (Davies 1996)

Old professionalism	New professionalism
Mastery of knowledge	Reflective practice
Unilateral decision process (Patient as dependent, colleagues as deferential)	Interdependent decision process (Patient as empowered, colleagues as involved)
Autonomy and self-management	Supported practice
Individual accountability	Collective responsibility
Detachment	Engagement
Specificity of practitioners' strengths	Inter-changeability of practitioners

need to develop a sense of shared responsibility for the overall management of the healthcare system, as well as for clinical practice with individual patients.

As this report has suggested, elements of the new professionalism are already beginning to emerge. All professional codes of conduct now espouse the value of team-working. An over-arching body, the Council for the Regulation of Healthcare Professions, is being given responsibility for overseeing and co-ordinating the work of the other regulatory bodies. Inter-professional education is beginning to be explored at an undergraduate level and is also being established as part of the continual professional development of registered professionals in some parts of the country. A new job evaluation framework has been developed to form the basis of NHS pay negotiations for non-medical staff (*Agenda for Change*).

However, other changes will be necessary if the new professionalism is to be effectively embedded across the workforce. The following section outlines a series of recommendations where further action is required.

Transforming training

New skills

The evidence and analysis set out in this report suggests that future health workers will need a range of skills in order to deliver genuinely patient centred care. These include the ability to:

- identify errors and hazards in care and to implement basic safety design principles in their practice (Institute of Medicine 2000)

- understand how to find new knowledge as it continually expands and to incorporate this knowledge into practice (Institute of Medicine 2001)

- know the root causes of ill health and disease, and the relationship between an individual's patients needs those of the wider community (Bissell and Jesson 2002).

- understand patients emotional and social needs as well as their physical and medical ones, and the process of care outside the hospital or primary care centre (Wistow 2002)

- work collaboratively in teams, with shared responsibilities for patient care (Kennedy *et al* 2001)

- adopt a shared decision making approach to patient professional interactions, for those patients who want it (Coulter 2001);

- explain and communicate the risks as well as benefits of different interventions; and support patients to take appropriate responsibilities for their own health and care, including how to self-care for minor conditions and self-manage long term illnesses (Kendall 2001)

- use a variety of approaches to deliver care, including the provision of care without face to face visits, for example using information technology to provide follow up care and routine monitoring (Wyatt 2002)

- understand managers' roles and the contribution they make to patient care, rather than solely focus on the individual clinical intervention (Harrison and Dixon 2000).

The need for future health workers to gain these skills raises important questions about the overall content of professional education. Training programmes have already undergone changes in recent decades. However, many commentators argue that the underlying experiences of educators and students have not been substantially altered. The medical curriculum has come under particular criticisms for being overcrowded and relying too much on memorising facts (Ludmerer 1999). A lack of funding to review and implement changes in the curriculum, the emphasis on research and patient care with little reward for teaching, the decentralised structure of medical schools and the presence of powerful departmental chairs, the fragmented responsibilities for different parts of the education system and the difficulties in assessing the impact of changes in teaching methods or curriculum have all been cited as reasons for the lack of genuine reform (Institute of Medicine 2001).

However, it is vital that a shared vision for health education in the 21st century is now developed. A major review of the content of the education system across undergraduate, graduate and continuing education for medical, nursing and other practitioners' training programmes should now be initiated to ensure that the future health workforce is able to deliver all of the elements that are integral to the delivery of high quality, patient-centred care.

Learning together

The ability of health practitioners to work together collaboratively is critical to delivering patient-centred care. Effective teamwork requires an education system which helps to foster understanding between all those entering the health workforce. This process must begin at the earliest stage: 'It is in the formative years of undergraduate education that attitudes are forged and skills imparted which shape the quality of engagement with patients for years to come' (Kennedy *et al* 2001). This has not been the hallmark of traditional professional education to date. Universities have for the most part educated those entering the professions in isolation from one another, with nursing and medical schools in many parts of the country emerging as geographically and organisationally separate institutions.

However, following the Bristol Royal Infirmary Inquiry, the Government committed itself to establishing common learning in all pre-registration programmes in England by 2004 (Department of Health 2001b). A set of common competencies that all practitioners should possess have been identified, such as communication skills and education about the principles and organisation of the NHS. There are already calls for this set of skills to be broadened to include some of the new skills necessary for delivering patient centred care which have been outlined above. For example, Salvage (2002) argues that common skills should include an understanding of different models of health and illnesses, including epidemiology, health and illness behaviour, health promotion and public health; emotional literacy, to aid closer working with patients; and the process of team working.

A number of barriers to the successful implementation of inter-professional training have already been identified. Perhaps the most important is the lack of evidence about its effectiveness. As Barr *et al* (2000) note in their review of the developing evidence base: 'Persuasive though arguments in favour of inter-professional education may be, evidence to substantiate them is elusive'. So for example, whilst the evidence that the greater the integration of inter-professional education into the wider curriculum the more positive the effect on attitudes to inter-professional collaborative working (Barnes *et al* 200), few studies provide evidence on longer-term outcomes. Crucially, most evaluations have been more concerned with student satisfaction than meeting external requirements (Barr *et al* 2000). However, as Humphris and Macleod Clark argue (2002) 'The dilemma simply put is that without innovation evidence cannot be developed...the mantra of the "evidence-base" could potentially become a constraint to the innovation necessary to address the significant workforce challenges faced by the future of health and social care'. More investment in evaluating inter-professional learning must be provided in future.

Inter-professional training may also require a shift in focus towards more training being delivered in practice. There is some evidence that practice-based inter-professional learning is more effective than theory based training in improving patient outcomes, such as satisfaction rates, and improving organisational outcomes such as positive behaviour amongst staff (Freeth *et al* 2001; Koppel and Reeves 2001). Workforce Development Confederations must work with universities to develop appropriate work-based learning. This should be supported through a system of fair reward for staff who support work-based learning, linked to incentives, appraisal and performance assessment (Humphris and Macleod Clark 2002).

There are also important practical barriers to inter-professional learning. These include the imbalance in student numbers between the different professions: an estimated 20,000 nurses entered training in 2000/1 compared to 4,300 medical student, 1,500 physiotherapists and 1,400 occupational therapists (Hale 2002). There are also widely different entry gates into the different professions – from NVQs to A grade A levels – and substantial difficulties in timetabling in a variety of programmes (Pirrie *et al* 1998). In addition, not all medical, nursing and other schools are located in the same site. There is considerable scepticism about whether the effort required to overcome practical barriers is justified when the ends of inter-professional education (encouraging collaborative working in order to improve the delivery of patient care) remain unproven (Hale 2002).

However, more fundamental concerns about the purpose of inter-professional training often underlie concerns about its purported practicality or otherwise. Some nurses fear the real agenda being pursued is not inter-professional training, where the professions learn together whilst remaining separate, but 'generic' training, which aims to create new practitioners along the lines proposed by the Future Healthcare Workforce Group. This, some critics believe, would ultimately lead to the deconstruction of the professions as part of an overall strategy to cut costs and jobs (Hale 2002). Despite reassurances from those engaged in implementing inter-professional learning programmes (Humphris and Macleod Clark 2002), many nurses remain deeply concerned about their purpose and goal.

The new practitioners proposed by the Future Healthcare Workforce Group are, however, being piloted at Kingston Hospital. Existing staff (that is, those who have already qualified) are being trained to become new Health Care Practitioners (who combine the skills of nurses, allied health professionals and doctors in training) and Health Care Practitioner Assistants (incorporating the roles of health care assistants, nursing auxiliaries and assistants and helpers to allied health professionals). The project is being evaluated and, if successful, may lead to a direct entry training point being developed for new staff. A key issue will be to embed sufficient choice in the system: if an individual initially chooses to train as a Health Care Practitioner but later decides they would rather be a nurse, physiotherapist or doctor, s/he should be able to change without having to start their training all over again.

An important issue underlying debates about the development of new practitioners like those being piloted at Kingston (and the related question of whether there should be generic or direct entry training) is the role that professional identity plays in encouraging people to enter the professions and in shaping the subsequent cultures and working practices of staff. Some commentators argue that people have a very clear idea of what sort of health worker they want to be when they embark on their training and that it will be far harder to attract people to train as a Health Care Practitioner than as a doctor, nurse or physiotherapist. Others point to evidence that a strong sense of professional identity can improve outcomes for patients, since it is associated with good teamwork and morale, and that a loss of professional identity can result in reductions in the quality of care (National Primary Care Research and Development Centre 1997).

However there is a strong argument, put forward by the Future Healthcare Workforce Group amongst others, that it is only by developing new types of practitioners who work across traditional professional divides and who focus on restoring health and well being as well as treating ill health, that outcomes for patients will be improved. Careful evaluations of the work being conducted at Kingston Hospital, and the piloting of new roles in other settings particularly primary care and across the health and social care sectors (see also below) will therefore be critical in determining how far this approach can and should be pursued in future.

New role models

It is important to remember that practitioners do not learn in higher education institutions alone. A large part of medical training, particularly post-graduate training, is based around apprenticeship. Role models play a hugely important role in shaping the working practices, cultures and attitudes of staff. The power of role models means incoming members of a profession have tended to adopt an identity similar to that of their mentors, perpetuating the profession as it is or as it was, rather than how it needs to be.

In future, role models must appreciate the differences between the values and approaches they were taught, and those required of new practitioners. Revalidation should play an important role in helping to change attitudes and perceptions. New types of role models also need to emerge. Role models and mentors need not necessarily be sought from within the same profession. Opportunities for doctors in training to learn from other practitioners, such as nurses and allied health professionals, should therefore be explored in future.

Improving training for the non-professionally qualified workforce

This report has emphasised the key role that non-professionally qualified staff already play in the process of patient care and suggested that their role is likely to expand in future. However, the needs of this section of the workforce have not been given sufficient priority to date. The lack of training support is a particular cause for concern: 80 per cent of social care staff and 38 per cent of NHS staff currently have no direct qualification, professional or vocational. There are currently very few in-service, part time, work-based courses that are open to the non-professionally qualified workforce. The norm is for Health Care Assistants and others to be seconded to full time courses within Higher Education. The NHSU should therefore make the expansion of part-time work-based routes into professional education a priority (Rogers 2002).

Making the skills escalator a reality

The development of the 'skills escalator' within the NHS, and its links to a reformed system of pay for non-medical staff through *Agenda for Change*, is a hugely welcome step. However, Rogers argues (2002) 'If the skills escalator is to be more than rhetoric, it must be possible for an HCA to do a shortened form of nurse education and to proceed eventually into medical education.'

It has been suggested that one of the obstacles to this progression is the fact that vocational and professional competencies are expressed in very different ways. NVQs are based on National Occupational Standards; professional qualifications are generally not. Without a common language of competence, it is argued, transition from support worker to professional (or 'from porter to doctor') is more difficult than it need be (Rogers 2002).

There have been calls for professional qualifications to be based on National Occupational Standards (NOSs). The use of occupational standards in professional areas like public health and social work are cited as evidence that this approach would also be possible for health professionals. Advocates acknowledge that NOSs would have to be reformed to remove the arcane language and perceived bureaucracy of the awarding bodies which have been a major cause of health professionals' resistance to using NOSs to date. Those who oppose argue that NOSs can never truly reflect the complexity of the work of health professionals or recognise the knowledge and expertise that underpins tasks.

If the skills escalator is to become a reality and if staff are really to receive equal pay for equal work (also see section on pay below), then there is a case for exploring whether professional qualifications could be based on NOSs over the longer term. NOSs for all health and social care qualifications below professional level are currently being reviewed and assessing whether it is possible to sufficiently reform NOSs remains a crucial question. In the meanwhile, greater encouragement and investment for accelerated training courses for health care assistants who want to become nurses and for experienced nurses who are seeking to become doctors should be provided.

It has been suggested that finding different points of entry into the professions and 'crediting in' people who have relevant experience could play an important role in helping to improve relationships between different professional groups (Murdock 2002; Vaughan 2002). One option would be to develop a national Credit Accumulation and Transfer Scheme, to work across the health and social care sectors, something which could be taken forward by the NHSU. Making participation a condition of the award of NHS education contracts – a major source of income for many universities – could help ensure high levels of uptake and compliance (Rogers 2002).

Creating a culture of innovation: new roles and new practitioners

In many quarters, the prevailing view is that reforming working practices primarily involves 'delegating' more of doctors' responsibilities to nurses. The evidence outlined in this report demonstrates that expanding nurses' roles has made a significant contribution to improving the quality of patient care. However, new roles and responsibilities for other members of the health team, and the potential for new types of practitioners, should be explored in future. There is a particular need to focus on primary care and the health and social care interface, since greater attention has so far tended to be paid to changing roles in acute care.

At the primary care level, pharmacists could become responsible for managing the medicines of patients with long term conditions, as well as monitoring patients' health status, checking for adverse drug reactions and screening for previously undiagnosed conditions. Expanding pharmacists' responsibilities may require the current role of pharmacist to be split in two: creating a consultant pharmacist (who would be responsible for medicines management and monitoring and screening patients) and a pharmacy technician (responsible for routine dispensing) (Murdock 2002).

Other new types of practitioners could emerge in primary care. For example, new 'information brokers' could be developed to provide patients with information about their conditions and diseases. These would be drawn from within the existing health workforce or be members of the local community who are given effective support and training (Pyper 2002).

New practitioners are also likely to emerge to help bridge the primary and secondary care divide. The need to provide seamless and integrated care for older people and to provide more care closer to home rather than in acute settings, suggests the need for a new practitioner focused on restoring and promoting health and independence. Intermediate care practitioners, who would combine elements of current professions such as nursing, occupational therapy and home support, could play an important role in addressing the needs of the 29 per cent of people who currently occupy acute hospital beds who do not need that level of care (Vaughan 2002).

New practitioners are also likely to be developed at the secondary care level. There is increasing interest in the potential for new physician assistants (Royal College of Physicians 2001). Physician assistants have been used in the US over the past 30 years. They are fully trained professionals who take on a role equivalent to that of a junior doctor for their entire career. Their responsibilities include assessing the patient's condition; conducting physical examinations, assessments, and diagnostic tests; developing treatment plans and admitting and discharging patients. In America, physician assistants work in all branches of medicine and surgery, have the ability to move to and from various clinical settings, have their own re-certification processes and do not compete for senior medical posts. Half of all physician assistants work in primary care; others work in emergency care, surgery, orthopaedics and other specialities (Hutchinson et al 2001).

The US experience of physician assistants raises some important issues when assessing their potential introduction to the UK. Studies of the use of physicians assistants in the US have shown they can provide quicker access to appointments, more attention to patients and better follow up care (Employing Doctors and Dentists 2000). However, they have not reduced unnecessary duplication of tasks at the level of the patient (for example with nursing) or improved the co-ordination of care between services (Hutchinson et al 2001). Inter-professional rivalries have in some cases been exacerbated by the use of physician assistants: in one US state nurses have actually prevented their introduction (Employing Doctors and Dentists 2000). A key lesson from the US is that physician assistants may attract those who want to provide medical care to patients but who do not want to go through (or who have failed to be accepted for) seven years of medical school, since their training takes two years. However, it is not yet clear whether the introduction of another healthcare career pathway in the UK would attract people into the health service who would not have joined professions with poor recruitment (Hutchinson *et al* 2001).

The role of the Health Care Practitioner, suggested by the Future Healthcare Workforce Group, has many similarities with that of the physician assistant. However, the key difference is that Health Care Practitioners are based on a social rather than medical model of health. HCPs also incorporate elements of nursing and physiotherapy, which the physician assistant role does not: a key issue at Kingston Hospital since it is the delays in providing physiotherapy for patients that is often a critical issue. As Hutchinson *et al* suggest (2001) the best way forward may therefore be to incorporate the aspects of the physician assistant system into local initiatives rather than implement a comprehensive national programme to train and employ US-style physician assistants across the board.

Implications for government and professional bodies

The Government's role in encouraging new roles and responsibilities must be to identify and remove any barriers to change at the local level, rather than attempt to impose new types of practitioners from the centre. The Department of Health has recognised the need to encourage innovation from the bottom up, in particular through the work of its Changing Workforce Programme. The Programme is supporting the piloting of a wide range of new roles, for example working with the Royal College of Physicians to see whether developing the role of medical secretaries could fill the non-clinical roles of physicians assistants and with the relevant Colleges to assess the potential for developing non-medical roles in the anaesthetic team, in part to help reduce doctors' working hours. Pilot programmes are also set to explore the potential to expand the role of surgical assistants to undertake minor surgical interventions.

However, more attention must now be paid to removing blocks to further innovation. Two overarching issues should be addressed. The first is to provide greater clarity about the Government's intentions for reforming the health workforce. This does not mean producing a detailed blueprint for reform, but rather that the Government should avoid giving out mixed messages about its strategy. The Government has emphasised the need to 'break down unnecessary professional demarcations' and explore the potential for new types of practitioners to emerge. Yet at the same time, it has pledged to provide an extra 7,500 consultants, 2,000 GPs, 20,000 nurses and 6,500 therapists: in other words 'more of the same'. These targets have a knock on effect throughout the system, driving workforce planning, how universities are monitored and how services are performance managed.

The second over-arching issue, related to the first, is the need to tackle 'the permission culture' in the NHS. Local NHS Trusts often feel they cannot be innovative without securing prior permission, either from their Strategic Health Authority or the Department of Health. So whilst staff have been trained to take on new roles and responsibilities, they may be unable to put these skills into practice because their employing organisation is unable or unwilling to work in new ways. Whilst it is true that the Government has committed itself to devolving and decentralising power within the health service, in order to encourage local innovation, there remains a very clear line of control from the Secretary of State, through the Chief Executive of the NHS and Department of Health, through to Chief Executives of NHS Trusts and Strategic Health Authorities. This line of control is a key factor underlying 'the permission culture' and will need to be tackled if Trusts are to feel more confident in experimenting with new ways of working.

A range of other issues will need to be addressed by central Government in order to create a culture of innovation. The way practitioners are paid can prevent them from taking on new roles. For example, the existing system for paying pharmacists mainly provides for the physical dispensing of prescriptions rather than broader roles such as screening for conditions or advising patients about how to self-care. This issue must be tackled if pharmacists are to fully contribute to the delivery of patient-centred care in future (Murdock 2002). (The issue of pay is returned to below.) There are also legal and practical barriers to change. Evaluations of nurse-led PMS pilots suggest nurses' restricted powers of certification and prescribing rights, and the inability of patients to register directly with nurses will need to be addressed if nurse roles are to further develop in future (Lewis 2001).

However, the experience of implementing new roles suggests there are also cultural and 'mythical' barriers to change. As Vaughan argues (2002): 'To a large extent the workforce has become disabled by its own presumptions...the division of labour...has developed through time and practice rather than any more logical reason but is deemed by practitioners and managers to be unalterable'. For example, since the publication of Scope of Professional Practice in 1992, nurses have been able to undertake a wide variety of tasks for which they have been judged competent. Yet misunderstandings based on past restrictions remain, with nurses unsure whether they are able to write sick notes or to assess patients themselves before referring them on. Local insight and variations in interpretations of the restrictions on different occupational groups are widespread.

Professional organisations have a critical role to play in tackling such cultural barriers to reform. The Royal Colleges should publicise evidence about emerging new roles and inform members who are interested in developing them where any legal barriers to change exist and when the barriers are more about custom and practice. Regulatory bodies will also need to provide greater clarity about competencies, training and quality assurance for new roles as and when they develop.

The future of regulation

Self-regulation has traditionally enshrined the assumption that only members of one's own profession are able to make a judgement on professional conduct. Regulatory bodies have already acknowledged the need to open their internal working processes up to patients and other members of the health team. An overarching body, the Council for the Regulation of Healthcare Professions, is also being established from April 2003. Its aim is to work with the existing regulatory bodies to build and manage a new framework for self-regulation which explicitly puts patients' interests first. The Council will enable co-ordination between the regulatory bodies and help share good practice and information. The Council is independent from government and directly answerable to Parliament. Whilst its aim is not to get involved with the direct regulation of health professionals, it will have the power to refer unduly lenient decisions about professionals' fitness to practice to the High Court.

It has been argued that co-regulation, rather than self-regulation, should become the guiding force of professional regulation in future. Since professionals have to work in partnership with each other, as well as with patients, a standard of good practice which covers all professionals should be developed (cited in Smith Institute 2002). This is something the Council for the Regulation of Healthcare Professionals could be responsible for drawing up in future.

The emergence of new roles presents challenges to the current regulatory environment. There is no established way for the regulatory system to respond to practitioners who are extending their scope of practice or attempting to work across professional 'silos', or where new roles are being developed for which there may be no pre-existing professionals to provide the necessary scrutiny. It will become increasingly difficult for uni-professional regulatory bodies to keep pace with emerging roles that require a wide range of competences, particularly where these competencies are not just associated with one profession. The role of the Council for the Regulation of Healthcare Professions in this process so far remains unclear. The Council must be empowered to manage a framework of self-regulation that can accommodate new and emerging roles which work across traditional professional divides, including the boundaries between health and social care.

The need for regulatory bodies to ensure the continuing competency of professionals has already been acknowledged by the medical profession: revalidation and appraisal for all doctors is being carried forward by the GMC. However, a number of important questions about ensuring the continuing competency of health professions remain. For example, should the recommendations for explicit codes of practice and revalidation put forward in the report of the Bristol Royal Infirmary Inquiry be applied to other professionals such as nurses and pharmacists?

An even more proactive approach to improving standards within the medical profession may be required in future, particularly in the light of an increasingly informed and less deferential public. The ex-president of the GMC, Sir Donald Irvine, has argued that the GMC and the Royal Colleges must shift their focus from ensuring minimum standards to guaranteeing optimal standards. This, he argues, 'will involve a huge change in outlook, practice and investment' and that despite the progress in revalidation and performance procedures 'there is unfinished business here' (Irvine 2002). The potential for the revalidation process to help change the working practices, cultures and attitudes of existing staff has yet to be fully explored and is a key challenge facing the professional bodies.

Another option for ensuring the continued competence of health professions has been suggested in the US. The Pew Health Professions Commission has argued that an additional level of oversight could be developed in which teams of practitioners, in addition to individuals, could be licensed or certified to perform certain tasks. For example, an individual receiving care for diabetes could go to a certified diabetes team that would ensure specific competencies and resources within that team. The certification requirements could be used as a measure of quality by patients and as a tool for quality improvement by teams seeking to obtain such certification (Institute of Medicine 2001).

Patient safety and improving standards are likely to remain a key issue for policy makers, practitioners and the public. In future, it will be anathema for key members of the health team to be entirely un-regulated as is currently the case for non-professionally qualified staff like health care assistants, particularly if their roles are set to increase. The Government has indicated its willingness to address this issue, however so far no actual changes have occurred in relation to the regulation of non-professionally staff. A number of different options have been put forward. These range from light touch approaches such as a code of practice or a negative register recording only those who have caused harm or may be likely to do so, to a more substantial options including a record of competencies or a register of approved workers (Johnson *et al* 2002). The Government must now consider these options as a matter of urgency.

An inclusive and fair system of pay

Health workers' pay has traditionally been negotiated nationally though a process of annual appeals by organisations representing each of the different occupational groups. Some significant changes to this process have been made in recent years. The most important of these is the development of a job evaluation framework to form the basis of pay negotiations for non-medical staff. *Agenda for Change* seeks to ensure practitioners are appropriately paid for taking on new roles and responsibilities and given 'equal pay for work of equal value'. However, doctors have not been part of this process. Their roles are not part of the job evaluation framework and they continue to conduct separate negotiations with Government over their terms and conditions. This could lead to problems in establishing a fair system of pay for nurses who have already taken on roles traditionally conducted by doctors, as well as for any attempts to further expand roles in future. The separation of negotiations for doctors' terms and conditions, and their disconnection from the pay scales of other professions through *Agenda for Change*, should be reviewed in future.

Over the longer term reducing disparities in pay between those working in health and social care will need to be tackled in order to facilitate the development of new roles and practitioners that work across traditional health and social care divides.

Improving workforce planning

The Government has acknowledged deep rooted problems with workforce planning in the NHS (Department of Health 2000c) and that workforce planning and service planning at a local level should be linked with workforce plans developed on a multi-disciplinary basis, looking across primary, secondary and tertiary care. In 2001, 27 new Workforce Development Confederations were established to manage education and training for the entire NHS workforce with a budget of nearly £3 billion. A National Workforce Development Board was also established, supported by a number of Care Group Workforce Teams which cover the priority areas of National Service Frameworks: mental health, cancer services, coronary heart disease, children's services and services for older people.

Workforce Development Confederations have made considerable progress to date, particularly in developing new forms of training that both widen entry into the professions and pioneer ways of improving practitioners' generic skills. WDCs are now being brought into Strategic Health Authorities to help strengthen their influence on strategic planning.

However, workforce planning is still based on the process of identifying gaps in the number of existing practitioners, rather than on assessing what types of practitioners with which sorts of skills are needed to meet the needs of the local population now and in future. Universities contracts with the NHS follow similar lines, with the main measures for monitoring universities focusing on quantity measures (such as the number of students being educated, attrition rates and how many qualify at the end) rather than on quality measures.

The Institute of Medicine has argued (2001) that: 'The starting point for addressing workforce issues should not be the present environment of licensure, reimbursement and organisation of care but a vision of how care ought to delivered in the 21st century'. Workforce planning must shift from determining the supply of clinicians in specific disciplines who continue to perform the same tasks using the same methods toward assessing the adequacy of supply given that future healthcare services will be based on providing continuous support through multidisciplinary approaches using modern technological support.

In particular, workforce planning must address the need to develop a workforce that can work across the health and social care divide. In future, there must be genuine integration of health and social care workforce planning and funding. An immediate option would be to pilot integrated workforce planning in some selected health economies (Humprhis and Macleod Clark 2002.)

System-wide changes

The need to ensure clinicians share responsibility for managing the process of reform has been a key theme in this report. Improving practitioners understanding of the role and contribution of managers, for example through specific modules in pre-registration training like those being used by St George's Medical School, will help deliver this goal.

However, the more fundamental challenge will be to effectively decentralise power and control within the NHS so that local clinicians and managers can work together to shape the way services are organised and delivered. A radical decentralisation of services may be critical in helping to tackle the 'permission culture' (outlined above) and encourage more innovative approaches to workforce reform, instead of focusing on protracted national negotiations between central government and professional organisations with all the political sensitivities these inevitably bring.

The Government has already recognised the need to cede power and resources to the 'front line'. *Shifting the Balance of Power* instituted a major reform of NHS structures, abolishing NHS Health Authorities and devolving 75 per cent of the NHS budget to Primary Care Trusts. However, many practitioners and managers have questioned the degree to which PCTs will be free to spend this money according to local priorities when the performance management process is predominantly geared towards delivering a series of hugely challenging national targets particularly around waiting times. In addition, whist politicians and managers may consider PCTs to be the 'front line', many clinicians feel professionals working at practice level are the real 'front line' of patient care, and that these clinicians are often disengaged from what happens even at the PCT level (cited in McLellan 2003).

Some policy makers and practitioners claim that genuine decentralisation will require other changes to the NHS. There has been growing interest in the potential for not-for-profit, mutual organisations to deliver health services (Maltby 2003; Lea and Mayo 2002; Commission on Public Private Partnerships 2002; Ham 1996). It has been argued that these organisations could help guarantee the freedom of local providers to shape the way care is provided and ensure both patients and staff are given a greater say over the way health services are run.

The Government has already proposed that the best performing hospital Trusts could become Foundation Hospitals: organisations which are independent from central government, and run by an elected Board of Governors including local users and members of staff. It has also signalled its intention that, over time, all Trusts could gain Foundation status.

There is currently much discussion of the merits or otherwise of Foundation Trusts. Several politicians and trades unions have argued that they will lead to a 'two-tier' health service and increase inequalities in access to care because of their proposed freedoms. Commentators have raised the problem of 'provider capture': that members of the public who are elected onto stakeholder councils may become cheerleaders for professional groups, choosing to retain and even enhance the services delivered by hospitals rather than ensuring they are delivered at the most appropriate level. Others argue that foundation status might be better applied to Primary Care Trusts, since it is as, if not more, important to ensure greater public and professional involvement over the process of commissioning health services as it is over their provision. There are also concerns from local government leaders that Foundation Trusts will cut across the accountability framework of local councils.

Foundation Trusts raise a series of difficult challenges that require careful attention, particularly the need to establish an appropriate balance between national standards and local control, and the importance of ensuring an effective and coherent framework of local accountability. However, the potential advantages of mutual organisations like Foundation Trusts, such as the role they could play in developing a greater sense of public and professional ownership over the management of services, and their ability to create a culture of innovation at the local level, suggests they should play an important role in the years ahead.

5. Conclusion

This report has argued that the working practices, cultures and attitudes of health practitioners are critical in determining the quality of care that patients receive. Whilst successive governments have talked about the need to reform the NHS workforce, their overwhelming political and policy focus has been on structural change. The current Government has not proved an exception to this rule.

Yet any government which seeks to improve the quality of care being provided must make reforming the health workforce a priority in future. This presents a particular challenge for progressive politicians and policy makers, who must seek to champion the invaluable contribution NHS staff make to delivering a more socially just society, whilst simultaneously questioning whether the roles, responsibilities and professional identities of these staff require fundamental reform.

The key to meeting this challenge is being clear about the overall objective of workforce or indeed any health policy reform: that of improving the quality of care being provided so that it better meets the needs of patients and improves patient outcomes. This goal is one that politicians, practitioners and patients alike can support and around which consensus for change can be built.

However in order to make this goal more than a superficial aspiration, a much clearer and more precise definition of what high quality, patient centred care is must be developed. Whilst the term 'patient-centred care' is frequently deployed, its precise meaning can differ widely according to who uses it. Professional bodies often automatically conflate their members' interests with those of patients, when this may not necessarily be the case. The Government's definition of patient-centred care is primarily about making access to services more timely and convenient and improving patients choices about where and when their operations take place. Whist these are certainly important features of a patient-centred system, they do not amount to a sufficiently broad or far sighted definition of the term.

The approach to patient-centred care set out in this book is based on an understanding of what patients want from their health services, but also on the evidence of what is necessary to deliver better patient outcomes, both now and in the future. Whilst many changes in working practices have taken place over recent decades, they have tended to focus on shorter term goals such as improving safety and making access to health services more timely and convenient. Far less attention has been paid to how workforce reforms could contribute to equally important characteristics of patient centred care such as informing and empowering patients. A particularly neglected issue is how the workforce will need to change in order to better promote health and wellbeing.

So more fundamental changes to the workforce will be necessary in order to deliver genuinely patient-centred care in future. Four main issues now face policy makers and practitioners: improving relations between clinicians and managers, ensuring closer working between practitioners and between sectors, transforming practitioner-patient relations and addressing the dominance of the medical model of health. These challenges have major implications for how the future health workforce should be planned, trained, paid and regulated. The Government's role in this process must be to identify and remove any barriers to local innovation rather than to impose a one-size-fits all vision from the centre. Embedding a culture of innovation within the NHS, to enable local services to develop new ways of working to meet local needs, must be a critical element of any future plans.

The impetus to seek imaginative solutions to the problems facing the NHS in general, and the health workforce in particular, could not be greater. We hope this report provides a useful contribution to the debate.

Endnotes

1 There is no satisfactory nomenclature for referring to the half a million people (headcount) who provide integral support services in the health service. To define staff by something they are not (ie 'non-professionally qualified') can be seen as demeaning (Rogers 2002). Likewise it may be considered inappropriate to refer to staff as 'non-registered' since there are persuasive arguments to suggest they should be. This section of the workforce has also been referred to as the 'support' workforce, although again this does not do justice to the degree of autonomous responsibility such staff often demonstrate (Thornley 1998).

2 Sir Roy Griffiths report of 1983 introduced the concept of general management to the NHS. Chantler (2002) points out that Griffiths did not actually intend to introduce a new profession of managers to the NHS and was clear that doctors needed to be closely involved in the management process. However this is not a widely acknowledged point.

3 Author's observations

4 The most high profile of these cases include children who received complex cardiac surgery at the Bristol Royal Infirmary, the misdiagnosis of cervical cytology at Kent and Canterbury, the poor and dangerous practice of the consultant Rodney Ledward and the murders committed by the GP Harold Shipman.

5 Cited by Sackett D, Perleth M and White K in 'The pre-history of evidence based healthcare' www.shef.ac.uk/~scharr/ir/percent.html

6 The term 'public health' has multiple meanings. It can be used to describe a *function*: public health science and the disciplines of epidemiology, health economics and medical statistics, traditionally carried out in public health departments by public health doctors. It can also be used to describe an *intervention*, which may be medical, such as screening or vaccination programmes, or focused on promoting health through changing individual lifestyle behaviour, such as campaigns to encourage people to exercise, eat healthily or stop smoking. Public health interventions also include community development, and action to engage communities and build social capital in order to improve health and well being. The new public health movement, which emerged in the 1980s, stressed the importance of understanding the underlying determinants of health,

such as poverty, unemployment and social exclusion, and the need to tackle these problems at both the national and community level.

7   The Future Healthcare Workforce Group has produced a series of bold reports on the future shape of the workforce for mental health, primary care, secondary acute care and care for the elderly. The Group's recommendations for secondary care are being piloted at Kingston Hospital NHS Trust in conjunction with St George's Hospital Medical School. These pilots are being supported by the Department of Health's Changing Workforce Programme and the Modernisation Agency.

8   The annual cost of treating the UK's 1.4 million diabetes patients is £5.2 billion (around nine per cent of the NHS budget). About 40 per cent of this goes on hospital care, yet a substantial proportion of this might be saved with more 'up-front' investment in prevention.

9   The evaluation will assess whether the new practitioners improve outcomes for patients compared to services provided by traditional professional groups (for example reducing waiting times for treatment and improving the co-ordination of care), as well as their impact on patient and staff satisfaction rates.

References

Adams C, Baeza J and Calnan M (2001) 'The new health promotion arrangements in general medical practice in England: Results from a national evaluation' *Health Education Journal* 60.1

Alberti G and Ham C (2002) 'The medical profession, the public and the government' *British Medical Journal* 324

Appleby J and Coote A (eds) (2002) *Five Year Health Check: A review of Government health policy 1997-2002* Kings Fund

Ashton J and Seymour H (1988) *The New Pubic Health* Open University Press

Audit Commission (1997) *The Coming of Age: Improving Care Services for Older People* Audit Commission

Audit Commission (1999) *Forget Me Not: Mental Health Services for Older People* Audit Commission

Audit Commission (2000) *The Way to Go Home: Rehabilitation and Remedial Services for Older People* Audit Commission

Audit Commission (2001) *Day Surgery: acute hospital portfolio: a review of national findings* Audit Commission

Audit Commission (2002) *Integrated services for older people: Building a whole system approach in England* Audit Commission

Balas A, Weingarten S and Garb C (2000) 'Improving Preventive Care by Prompting Physicians' *Archive of International Medicine* 160.3 cited in Institute of Medicine (2001) *Crossing the Quality Chasm: A New Health System for the 21st Century* National Academy Press

Barnes D, Carpenter J and Dickinson C (2000) 'Interprofessional education for community mental health: attitudes to community care and professional stereotypes' *Social Work Education* 19.6

Barr H, Freeth D, Hammick M, Koppel I and Reeves S (2000) *Evaluations of Interprofessional Education: A UK review for Health and Social Care* CAIPE/The British Educational Research Association

Black A and Garside P (1994) 'Health Management Guide: Patient-focused Care' *Health Service Journal* Supplement 23.6.94

Blenkinsopp A and Bradley C (1996) 'Patients, society and the increase of self-medication' *British Medical Journal* 312

Blissell P and Jesson J (200) 'Health Inequalities: a neglected area of pharmacy policy and practice' *Pharmaceutical Journal* 269.7227

Bloor K and Maynard A (2002) 'Consultants: managing them means measuring them' *Health Service Journal* 19.12.02

Blue L *et al* (2001) 'Radomised controlled trial of specialist nurse intervention in heart failure' *British Medical Journal* 323

Booth, A (2000) *What proportion of healthcare is evidence based? Resource Guide* School of Health and Related Research, University of Sheffield www.shef.ac.uk/~scharr/ir/percent.html

British Medical Association (2002) *A New Model for NHS Care* Health Policy and Economic Research Unit Discussion Paper 9 BMA

Cabinet Office (2000) *Delivery of Public Services, 24 Hours a Day, Seven Days a week (24x7)* People's Panel TSO

Cassileth B, Zupkis R, Sutton-Smith K and March V (1980) 'Information and participation preferences among cancer patients' *Annuls of Internal Medicine* 92

Chantler C (2002) 'The second greatest benefit to mankind?' *The Lancet* 360

Chapple A, Rogers A, Macdonald W and Sergison M (2000) 'Patients perceptions of changing professional boundaries and the future of nurse led services' *Primary Health Care Research and Development* 1

Clark N and Gong M (2000) 'Management of chronic disease by practitioners and patients: are we teaching the wrong things?' *British Medical Journal* 320

Cochrane D *et al* (2002) *The Future Healthcare Workforce: the third report* Chamberlain Dunn Associates

Cochrane D *et al* (1999) *The Future Healthcare Workforce: the second report* Bournemouth University

Commission on Public Private Partnerships (2002) *Building Better Partnerships: The final report of the Commission on Public Private Partnerships* ippr

Cooper J (2001a) *Partnerships for Successful Self-Management: The Living with Long-term Illness (Lill) Project Report* Long-term Medical Conditions Alliance

Cooper M (2001b) *An evaluation of the safety and effectiveness of the emergency nurse practitioner in the treatment of patients with minor injuries: a pilot study* Glasgow Royal Infirmary

Coronary Heart Disease Collaborative (2001) www.nhs.uk/npat

Cotton M, Bucknall C, Dagg K and Johnson M (2000) 'Early hospital discharge for exacerbation of chronic obstructive pulmonary disease: A randomised controlled trial' *Thorax* 55

Coulter A (2002) *The Autonomous Patient: Ending paternalism in medical care* TSO

Coulter A, Entwistle V and Gilbert D (1999) 'Sharing decisions with patients: is the information good enough?' *British Medical Journal* 318

Coulter A and Cleary P (2001) 'Patients' experiences with hospital care in five countries' *Health Affairs* 20

Curley A, McClure G, Spence D and Craig S (2003) 'What new NHS?' *Health Service Journal* 23.1.03

Darzi A (1999) 'Wedded Bliss?' *Health Service Journal* 10.6.99

Davidoff F, Haynes B, Sackett D and Smith R (1995) *British Medical Journal* 310

Davies A (2002) 'Structures and Accountability' in Kendall L and Harker L (eds) (2002) *From Wellfare to Wellbeing: the future of social care* ippr

Davies C (1996) 'A new vision of professionalisms' *Nursing Times* 92

Davies C (1999) 'Doctors and Nurses: changing family values?' *British Medical Journal* 319

Davies L, Wilkinson M, Bonner S, Cleverley P and Angus R (1999) 'A randomised controlled trial of home care (ACTRITE) versus hospital admission in exacerbations of chronic obstructive pulmonary disease (COPD)' *Eur Respir J* 14, suppl 3 387

Davis D, Thomson M, Oxman A and Haynes B (1995) 'Changing Physician Performance: A Systematic Review of the Effect of Continuing Medical Education Strategies' *JAMA* 274 cited in Institute of Medicine (2001) *Crossing the Quality Chasm: A New Health System for the 21st Century* National Academy Press

Department of Health and Social Security (1986) *Mix and Match: A review of nursing skills mix* HMSO

Department of Health (2002a) *Vacancy survey 2002* www.doh.gov.uk/public/vacancysurvey.htm

Department of Health (2002b) *Public Sector Making a Difference* Regulatory Impact Unit TSO

Department of Health (2001a) *Building a safer NHS for patients* TSO

Department of Health (2001b) *Working Together – Learning Together. A lifelong learning framework for the NHS* TSO

Department of Health (2001c) *The report of the Chief Medical Officer's Project to Strengthen the Public Health Function* TSO

Department of Health (2000a) *The NHS Plan: A Plan for Investment – A Plan for Reform* TSO

Department of Health (2000b) *An Organisation with a Memory* TSO

Department of Health (2000c) *A Health Service of All the Talents: developing the NHS workforce* TSO

Department of Health (1998) *The National Survey of NHS Patients: General Practice*

Durieux P, Nizard R and Ravaud P (2000) 'A Clinical Decision Support System for Prevention of Venous Thromboembolism' *JAMA* 283 cited in Institute of Medicine (2001) *Crossing the Quality Chasm: A New Health System for the 21st Century* National Academy Press

Edwards L (2002) *The First Twelve Months: the parent perspective* ippr

Edwards L (2001) *The Future of Healthcare: the patient perspective in England* ippr

Edwards L and Clarke R (2001) *Quality and the NHS: the patient perspective* ippr

Ellis J, Mulligan I, Rowe J and Sackett D (1995) 'Inpatient general medicine is evidence based' *The Lancet* 345

Elwyn G, Edwards A, Kinnersley P, Grol R (2000) 'Shared decision making and the concept of equipoise: the competences of involving patients in healthcare choices' *British Journal of General Practice* 50

Employing Doctors and Dentists (2000) 'Is the future rosy for physicians assistants?' *Employing Doctors and Dentists* 26

Etzioni A (1969) *The Semi-professions and their Organization* Free Press

Evans R, Pestonik S and Classen D (1998) 'A Computer-Assisted Management Program for Antibiotics and other Anti-infective Agents' *New England Journal of Medicine* 338.4, cited in Institute of Medicine (2001) *Crossing the Quality Chasm: A New Health System for the 21st Century* National Academy Press

Evidence-Based Medicine Working Group (1992) 'Evidence Based Medicine: a New Approach to Teaching the Practice of Medicine' *JAMA* 268.17 cited in Institute of Medicine (2001) *Crossing the Quality Chasm: A New Health System for the 21st Century* National Academy Press

Fishwick S and Letts M (2002) 'The Lay Person as Healthcare Practitioner' in Lissauer R and Kendall L (eds) (2002) *New practitioners in the Future Health Service: exploring roles for practitioners in primary and intermediate care* ippr

Freeth D, Reeves S and Goreham C (2001) '"Real life" clinical learning on an interprofessional training ward' *Nurse Education Today* 21

Gerteis M, Edgman-Levitan S, Daley J, Delbanco T (1993) *Through the patients' eyes: understanding and promoting patient-centred care* Jossey Bass

Gill P, Dowell A, Neal R, Smith N, Heywood P and Wilson A (1996) 'Evidence based general practice: a retrospective study of interventions in one training practice' *British Medical Journal* 312

Gillespie R, Florin D and Gillam S (2002) *Changing Relationships – Findings of the Patient Involvement Project* The King's Fund

Greene A (1994) 'Performance, productivity, and managing costs: the successor to patient-focused care: hospital process re-engineering' *The Health Summary* xi (i)

Gollop R (2003) 'Modernisation: Fear of flying' *Health Service Journal* 23

Gowman N and Coote A (2000) *Evidence and Public Health: Towards a Common Framework* The King's Fund

Grol R, Wensing M, Mainz J, Rerreira P, Hearnshaw H and Hjortdah P (1999) 'Patients' priorities with respect to general practice care: an international comparison' *Family Practice* 16

Hale C (2002) *Questioning the Conventional Wisdom* www.ippr.org

Ham C (1996) *Public, private or community: what next for the NHS?* Demos

Han B and Haley WE (1998) 'Family Care giving for Patients with Stroke: Review and Analysis' *Stroke* 30.7 quoted in Robinson M (2002) *Moving on After a Stroke: A Structured Literature Review* Nuffield Institute for Health

Harker L and Kendall L (2003) *An Equal Start? Improving Support During Pregnancy and the First Twelve Months* ippr

Harrison A and Dixon J (2000) *The NHS: Facing the Future* The King's Fund

Hassell K, Whittington Z, Cantrill J, Bates F, Rogers A and Noyce P (2001) *Care at the Chemist: A Question of Access – a feasibility study comparing community pharmacy and general practice management of minor ailments* University of Manchester

Henwood M (2001) *Future Imperfect? Report of the King's Fund Care and Support Inquiry* The King's Fund

Horrocks S, Andeson E and Salisbury C (2002) 'Systematic review of whether nurse practitioners working in primary care can provide equivalent care to doctors' *British Medical Journal* 324

Humphris D and Macleod Clark J (2002) *Shaping a vision for a 'New Generation' workforce* www.ippr.org

Hutchinson L, Marks T and Pittilo M (2001) 'The physician assistant: would the US model meet the needs of the NHS?' *British Medical Journal* 323

Institute of Medicine (2001) *Crossing the Quality Chasm: A New Health System for the 21st Century* National Academy Press

Institute of Medicine (2000) *To Err is Human: Building a Safer Health System* National Academy Press

Irvine D (2002) *Patients, Doctors and the Public Interest* DARE Lecture given at the Faculty of Public Health Medicine's Annual Scientific Meeting, 27.6.02

Johnson M *et al* (2001) 'Hospital at home services for acute exacerbation of chronic obstructive pulmonary disease: a survey of British practice' *Health Bulletin* 59.3

Johnson M, Allsop J, Clark M, Davies C, Biggerstaff D, Genders N and Saks M (2002) *Regulation of Healthcare Assistants* www.ippr.org

Jones D (2000) 'Nurse-led PMS pilots' in Lewis R and Gillam S (2000) *Transforming Primary Care: Personal medical services in the new NHS* The King's Fund

Kaplan S, Gandek B, Greenfield S, Rogers W and Ware J (1995) 'Patient and visit characteristics related to physicians' participatory decision-making style: results from the medical outcomes study' *Med Care* 333

Kendall L (2001) *The Future Patient* ippr

Kendrick S (1994) 'The increase in the number of emergency admissions: age, diagnosis, frequency' (working paper for the acute beds research group) *Information and Statistics Division* NHSIS

Kennedy I *et al* (2001) *The Report of the Bristol Royal Infirmary Inquiry* TSO

Kinnersley P, Anderson E, Parry K, Clement J, Archard L, Turton P (2000) 'Randomised controlled trial of nurse practitioner versus general practitioner care for patients requesting 'same day' consultations in primary care'

Klein R (1993) *The politics of the National Health Service* Longman

Koppel I and Reeves S (2001) 'Establishing a systematic approach to evaluating the effectiveness of interprofessional education' *Issues in Interdisciplinary Care* 3.1

Lathrop P (1993) *Restructuring health care: the patient-focused paradigm* Jossey Bass

Lawrence D (2002) *Can the NHS learn from the USA? The Kaiser Permanente experience of integrated care* 9th Annual Office of Health Economics Lecture delivered by David Lawrence MD, Chairman and Chief Executive Officer of Kaiser Permanente

Lea R and Mayo E (2002) *The Mutual Health Service: how to decentralise the NHS* Institute of Directors and New Economics Foundation

Le Fanu J (1999) *The rise and fall of modern medicine* Little Brown and Company

Le Grand J (2003) 'Schooled in Success' *Health Service Journal* 16.1.03

Lenaghan J (1998) *Brave New NHS? The impact of the new genetics on the health service* ippr

Levenson R (1997) *Developing Public Health in the NHS: The Multi-disciplinary Function* The King's Fund

Lewis R (2001) *Nurse-led Primary Medical Services* Pilots The King's Fund

Lister G (2002) *Cost Drivers and Health Futures 2002-2022* (unpublished mimeo)

Ludmerer K (1999) *Time to Heal: American Medical Education from the Turn of the Century to the Era of Managed Care* Oxford University Press

Lyall J (2003) 'Modernisation: Alien concept' *Health Service Journal* 23.1.03

Maltby P (2003) *In the public interest? Assessing the potential of Public Interest Companies* ippr

Martin S (2002) 'Developing the nurse practitioner's role in minor surgery' *Nursing Times* 98.33

McClimont B (2002) 'The Home Care Workforce: Urgent Attention Required' *Building knowledge for integrated care* 10.4

McCoy K (2000) *Review of Care in the Community* Social Services Inspectorate, Department of Health, Social Services and Public Safety Northern Ireland

McKinsey and Company (2001) *Expectations of the 2020 UK Healthcare system* Health Trends Review: Proceedings of conference held at the Barbican Centre, London, 18-19.10.01

McLellan A (2003) 'Practice makes perfect: interview with National Association of Primary Care Chair, Dr Peter Smith' *Health Service Journal* 16.1.03

Moynihan R and Smith R (2002) 'Too much medicine?' *British Medical Journal* 324

Mudinger M, Kane R, Lenz E, Totten A, Tsasi W, Clearly P, Friedewald W, Siu A, Shelanshi M (2000) 'Primary care outcomes in patients treated by nurse practitioners or physicians' *JAMA* 283.1

Muir Gray J (1995) 'Post-modern medicine' *The Lancet* 354

Murdock A (2002) 'The Consultant Pharmacist and Pharmacist Technician in Primary Care' in Lissauer R and Kendall L (eds) (2002) *New Practitioners in the Future Health Service: exploring roles for practitioners in primary and intermediate care* ippr

Naish J (2002) *Health Inequalities and Children Under One: The Contribution of Health Services* www.ippr.org

National Consumer Council (1998) *Consumer concerns 1998: a consumer view of helath services: the report of an RSL survey* NCC

National Primary Care Research and Development Centre (1997) *Cultural differences between medicine and nursing: implications for primary care* NPCRDC, University of Manchester

New B (2000) *What Business is the NHS in? Establishing the boundary of a healthcare system's responsibility* ippr

NHSE (1996) *Progress with Patient – Focused Care in the UK* Nuffield Institute for Health

Nuffield Foundation (1986) *Pharmacy: The report of a committee of inquiry* Nuffield Foundation

Nursing and Midwifery Council (2002) *Code of Professional Conduct* Nursing and Midwifery Council

Pirrie A, Wilson V, Harden R and Elsegood J (198) 'AMEE Guide 12: Multiprofessional education: Part 2, Promoting cohesive practice in healthcare' *Medical Teacher* 20.5

Pyper C (2002) 'Knowledge brokers as change agents' in Lissauer R and Kendall L (eds) (2002) *New practitioners in the future health service: exploring roles for practitioners in primary and intermediate care* ippr

Ramprogus V and O'Brien D 'The case for the formal education of Health Care Assistants' in *Nursing Times* 98.27

Risk A and Dzenowagis J (2001) 'Review of internet health information quality initiatives' *Journal of Medical Internet Research* 3.4

Rivett G (1998) *From Cradle to Grave: Fifty years of the NHS* The King's Fund

Rogers A, Hassell K and Nicolaas G (1999) *Demanding patients? Analysing the Use of Primary Care* Open University Press

Rogers J (2002) *Support staff in health and social care – an overview of current policy issues* www.ippr.org

Rowe A (2002)'Using a 'whole systems' approach to change service delivery' *Community Practitioner* 74.3

Royal College of General Practitioners and the Faculty of Public Health Medicine (2001) *Public Health in the New NHS Structures: The Primary Care Perspective*

Royal College of Nursing (2002) *The community approach to improving public health: community nurses and community development* RCN

Royal College of Physicians (2001) *Skill-mix and the Hospital Doctor: New Roles for the Health Care Workforce* Royal College of Physicians

Royal College of Surgeons (2001) *The Surgical Workforce in the New NHS* Royal College of Surgeons

Rummery K and Glendinning C (2000) *Primary Care and Social Services: Developing New Partnerships for Older People* Radcliffe Medical Press

Sakr M, Angus J, Perrin J, Nixon C, Nicholl J, Wardrope J (1999) 'Care of minor injuries by emergency nurse practitioners or junior doctors: a randomised controlled trial' *The Lancet* 354

Salvage J (2002) *Rethinking Professionalism: The First Step for Patient Focused Care?* www.ippr.org

Sanderson D, Limber C, Eldret C and Harrison K (2003) 'To the ENT degree' *Health Service Journal* 27.2.03

Schofield M (1996) *The Future Healthcare Workforce: the Steering Group report* HSMU

Shea S, DuMouchel W and Bahamonde L (1996) 'A Meta-Analysis of 16 Randomised Controlled Trials to Evaluate Computer Based Clinical Reminder Systems for Preventive Care in the Ambulatory Setting' *JAMA* 3.6 cited in Institute of Medicine (2001) *Crossing the Quality Chasm: A New Health System for the 21st Century* National Academy Press

Shum C, Humphreys A, Wheeler D, Cochrane M, Skoda S, Clement S (2000) 'Nurse management of patients with minor illnesses in general practice: multi-centre, randomised controlled trial' *British Medical Journal* 320

Smith S, Roberts M, Balmer S (2000) 'Role Overlap and Professional Boundaries: Future Implications for Physiotherapy and Occupational Therapy in the NHS' *Physiotherapy* 8.6

Smith R (2002) 'Take back your mind, take back your pearls' *British Medical Journal* 325

Smith R (2001) 'Why are doctors so unhappy?' *British Medical Journal* 322

Smith Institute (2002) *Risk and Trust in the NHS* The Smith Institute

Stewart M (2001) 'Toward a global definition of patient centred care' *British Medical Journal* 322

Swarska E, Cohen G, Swrsk K, Lamb Q *et al* (2000) 'A randomised controlled trial of supported discharge in patient with exacerbations of chronic obstructive pulmonary disease' *Thorax* 55

Taylor D (2001) *Modernising Self Care: Relieving illness, reducing disability and promoting good health* Boots Health Briefing 1

Tennant R and Woodhead D (2002) 'The Public Health Leader' in Lissauer R and Kendall L (eds) (2002) *New practitioners in the future health service: exploring the roles for practitioners in primary and intermediate care* ippr

Thornley C (1998) *Neglected nurses, hidden work: an investigation into the pay and employment of nursing auxiliaries/assistants in the NHS* UNISON

Turner M (2000) 'It is what you do and the way that you do it: Service users views on the introduction of codes of conduct and practice for social care workers by the four national care councils' *Shaping Our Lives* National Institute for Social Work

Vaughan B (2002) 'The Intermediate Care Practitioner' in Lissauer R and Kendall L (eds) (2002) *New practitioners in the future health service: exploring roles for practitioners in primary and intermediate care* ippr

Vaughan B and Withers G (2002) 'Acute Distress' *Health Service Journal* 9.5.02

Vickery D and Lynch W (1995) 'Demand management: enabling patients to use medical care appropriately' *Journal of Occupational and Environmental Medicine* 7

Wade D (2003) 'Altered Egos' *Sunday Times Magazine* 12.1.03

Walker J, Brooksby A, McInerny J and Taylor A (1998) 'Patient perception of hospital care: building confidence, faith and trust' *Journal of Nursing Management* 6

Wanless D (2002) *Securing our Future Health: Taking a Long-Term View Final Report* TSO

Wanless D (2001) *Securing our Future Health: Taking a Long-Term View Interim Report* TSO

Wilkinson P *et al* (1997) 'A Long Term Follow Up of Stroke Patients' *Stroke* 28.3 quoted in Robinson M (2002) *Moving on After a Stroke: A Structured Literature Review* Nuffield Institute for Health

Williams S and Calnan M (1991) Key determinants of consumer satisfaction with general practice' *Family Practice* 8

Williams S, Weinman J and Dale J (1998) 'Doctor patient communication and patient satisfaction: a review' *Family Practice* 15

Williams S *et al* (2002) 'General practitioners with special clinical interests: a model for improving respiratory disease management' *British Journal of General Practice* 52.483

Wilson A, Pearson D and Hassey A (2002) 'Barriers to developing the nurse practitioner role in primary care: the GP perspective' *Family Practice* 19.6

Wistow G (2002) 'The future aims and objectives of social care' in Kendall L and Harker L (eds) (2002) *From Welfare to Wellbeing: The Future of Social Care* ippr

Wyatt J (2002) 'The Telecarer: a new role for clinical professionals' in Lissauer R and Kendall L (eds) (2002) *New practitioners in the future health service: exploring roles for practitioners in primary and intermediate care* ippr